Patient Assessment in Pharmacy

A Culturally Competent Approach

Edited by

Yolanda M. Hardy, PharmD

Associate Professor
College of Pharmacy
Chicago State University
Chicago, Illinois

W0008807

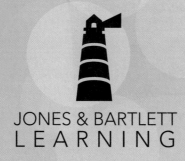

JONES & BARTLETT
LEARNING

World Headquarters
Jones & Bartlett Learning
5 Wall Street
Burlington, MA 01803
978-443-5000
info@jblearning.com
www.jblearning.com

Jones & Bartlett Learning books and products are available through most bookstores and online booksellers. To contact Jones & Bartlett Learning directly, call 800-832-0034, fax 978-443-8000, or visit our website, www.jblearning.com.

Substantial discounts on bulk quantities of Jones & Bartlett Learning publications are available to corporations, professional associations, and other qualified organizations. For details and specific discount information, contact the special sales department at Jones & Bartlett Learning via the above contact information or send an email to specialsales@jblearning.com.

Copyright © 2016 by Jones & Bartlett Learning, LLC, an Ascend Learning Company

All rights reserved. No part of the material protected by this copyright may be reproduced or utilized in any form, electronic or mechanical, including photocopying, recording, or by any information storage and retrieval system, without written permission from the copyright owner.

The content, statements, views, and opinions herein are the sole expression of the respective authors and not that of Jones & Bartlett Learning, LLC. Reference herein to any specific commercial product, process, or service by trade name, trademark, manufacturer, or otherwise does not constitute or imply its endorsement or recommendation by Jones & Bartlett Learning, LLC and such reference shall not be used for advertising or product endorsement purposes. All trademarks displayed are the trademarks of the parties noted herein. *Patient Assessment in Pharmacy: A Culturally Competent Approach* is an independent publication and has not been authorized, sponsored, or otherwise approved by the owners of the trademarks or service marks referenced in this product.

There may be images in this book that feature models; these models do not necessarily endorse, represent, or participate in the activities represented in the images. Any screenshots in this product are for educational and instructive purposes only. Any individuals and scenarios featured in the case studies throughout this product may be real or fictitious, but are used for instructional purposes only.

The authors, editor, and publisher have made every effort to provide accurate information. However, they are not responsible for errors, omissions, or for any outcomes related to the use of the contents of this book and take no responsibility for the use of the products and procedures described. Treatments and side effects described in this book may not be applicable to all people; likewise, some people may require a dose or experience a side effect that is not described herein. Drugs and medical devices are discussed that may have limited availability controlled by the Food and Drug Administration (FDA) for use only in a research study or clinical trial. Research, clinical practice, and government regulations often change the accepted standard in this field. When consideration is being given to use of any drug in the clinical setting, the health care provider or reader is responsible for determining FDA status of the drug, reading the package insert, and reviewing prescribing information for the most up-to-date recommendations on dose, precautions, and contraindications, and determining the appropriate usage for the product. This is especially important in the case of drugs that are new or seldom used.

9073-1

Production Credits

Chief Executive Officer: Ty Field
President: James Homer
Chief Product Officer: Eduardo Moura
Executive Editor: Rhonda Dearborn
Editorial Assistant: Sean Fabery
Associate Director of Production: Julie C. Bolduc
Production Assistant: Brooke Appe
Marketing Manager: Grace Richards
Art Development Editor: Joanna Lundeen
Art Development Assistant: Shannon Sheehan
VP, Manufacturing and Inventory Control: Therese Connell
Composition: Cenveo Publisher Services

Cover Design: Michael O'Donnell
Manager of Photo Research, Rights & Permissions: Amy Rathburn
Rights and Photo Research Coordinator: Mary Flatley
Cover Image: background, © antishock/ShutterStock, Inc.; doctor taking woman's blood pressure, © Tyler Olson/Shutterstock, Inc.; measuring blood sugar with a blood glucose meter, © Ververidis Vasilis/ Shutterstock, Inc.; doctor standing beside patient on weighing machine © bikeriderlondon/Shutterstock, Inc.
Printing and Binding: Courier Companies
Cover Printing: Courier Companies

Library of Congress Cataloging-in-Publication Data
Hardy, Yolanda, author.
    Patient assessment in pharmacy : a culturally competent approach / by Yolanda Hardy.
        p. ; cm.
    Includes bibliographical references and index.
    ISBN 978-1-284-02574-3 (pbk. : alk. paper)
    I. Title.
    [DNLM: 1. Cultural Competency—United States. 2. Pharmaceutical Services—United States. 3. Medical History Taking—United States. 4. Needs Assessment—United States. 5. Physical Examination—United States. 6. Professional-Patient Relations—United States. QV 21]
    RM301.12
    615.1—dc23
                                            2014014064

6048
Printed in the United States of America
18 17 16 15 14   10 9 8 7 6 5 4 3 2 1

Dedication

This book is dedicated to my patients. Thank you for allowing me to participate in the management of your care. I've learned something from each of you. You have inspired me and have helped me to become a better practitioner. Thank you.

Contents

Preface

With the increasing diversity of our patient population, the importance of achieving health equity in our healthcare system, the ever-increasing responsibility of the pharmacist as a provider of patient care, and my own experience as a patient and a provider of care, it seemed only natural that a book created to help prepare pharmacists for the provision of care to patients of different backgrounds was valuable and needed. Hence, this book—*Patient Assessment in Pharmacy: A Culturally Competent Approach*—was created. This book is intended to help pharmacy students, pharmacy residents, and practicing pharmacists learn not only how to properly assess patients, but also how to do so in a culturally appropriate manner. This book was designed using a practical and engaging approach to cover those topics that pharmacists can encounter at any time during practice.

I created this book in part to serve as a text for Patient Assessment or Physical Assessment courses in any level of the pharmacy curriculum. Students who are early in their pharmacy career can benefit from the use of this text because it provides them with key questions to ask in order to perform basic triage. Students who are further along in their pharmacy career can benefit from this book because it provides them with skills that can be integrated into therapeutics-based courses and practicum experiences.

Organization of the Text

This text is unique because it is organized in a manner that mirrors the approach to a patient visit. First, as practitioners, we prepare for the visit prior to seeing the patient. Once we see the patient, we typically begin with the patient interview, incorporating physical assessment techniques when appropriate. Last, we take into consideration all the information we have gathered and create our care plan.

The text is divided into four units that highlight each of these steps. Unit I, "Preparing for the Provision of Culturally Competent Pharmaceutical Care," readies the learner by discussing why culturally competent care is needed. In addition, this unit provides an overview of cultural competency models.

Unit II, "The Culturally Competent Patient Interview and History," discusses the process for conducting a patient history and interview with an emphasis on integrating explanatory models in order to gather the patient viewpoint on disease processes and management.

Unit III, "The Culturally Competent Physical Assessment," focuses on physical assessment as well as key interview questions that can help gather more culturally appropriate information from the patient. Each chapter in this unit focuses on an organ system and discusses common medical conditions that the pharmacist may encounter, with an emphasis on medical conditions that may be particular to certain cultures.

Each chapter includes a review of the clinical presentation of disease, questions to ask during the patient interview, and physical assessment techniques used to further assess the disease state. In addition, each chapter contains a review of the clinical presentation of drug-induced processes. Chapters in this unit end with a discussion on cultural considerations related to the assessment of disease processes.

The book brings these threads together in Unit IV, "The Culturally Competent Care Plan," which discusses how explanatory models can be used to help create the care plan.

Features and Benefits

To assist the learning process, each chapter begins with a list of objectives and key terms to focus student learning. Case studies and examples appear throughout the text to help learners apply the information they have just read. Numerous color photographs and illustrations accompany the text so that learners can familiarize themselves with how a disease, sign, or symptom may appear on persons with different skin tones. Finally, each chapter concludes with a series of review questions that the student can answer for self-study or as an assignment.

Instructor Resources

This text is accompanied by ancillary materials that will aid in the teaching and learning process. These materials are designed to reinforce concepts learned from the textbook. Instructor materials include:

- Test Bank, including more than 300 questions
- Instructor's Manual, containing Lab Worksheets, Sample Syllabus, and an Answer Key for end-of-chapter Review Questions
- Lecture Outlines in PowerPoint format, featuring more than 350 slides

Acknowledgments

It was an exciting journey writing this book, and it is my hope that you will find this book informative and enjoyable. I would like to thank all of the contributing authors who shared the vision for creating this text—it certainly would not have been possible without your dedication and expertise! I would also like to thank the students, faculty, and staff at Chicago State University College of Pharmacy for being supportive and inspirational during this process. Last, I would like to thank my family for being patient and supportive during this endeavor, especially my nephew, who told me to make sure that the "book isn't boring."

Contributors

Carmita A. Coleman, PharmD, MAA
Associate Dean
College of Pharmacy
Chicago State University
Chicago, Illinois

Heather Fields, PharmD, MPH, BCACP
Assistant Professor
College of Pharmacy
Chicago State University
Chicago, Illinois

Antoine T. Jenkins, PharmD, BCPS
Assistant Professor
College of Pharmacy
Chicago State University
Chicago, Illinois

Charisse Johnson, MS, PharmD
Director of the Office of Experiential
    Education
College of Pharmacy
Chicago State University
Chicago, Illinois

Janene L. Marshall, PharmD, BCPS
Assistant Professor
College of Pharmacy
Chicago State University
Chicago, Illinois

Mark D. Watanabe, PharmD, PhD, BCPP
Assistant Clinical Professor
School of Pharmacy
Northeastern University
Boston, Massachusetts

Reviewers

Michael A. Biddle, Jr., PharmD, BCPS
Assistant Professor
Albany College of Pharmacy and Health
    Sciences, Vermont
Colchester, Vermont

Beth Buckley, PharmD, CDE
Assistant Professor
School of Pharmacy
Concordia University, Wisconsin
Mequon, Wisconsin

Lakesha M. Butler, PharmD, BCPS
Clinical Associate Professor
Edwardsville School of Pharmacy
Southern Illinois University
Edwardsville, Illinois

Krista D. Capehart, PharmD, MSPharm
Associate Professor
School of Pharmacy
University of Charleston
Charleston, West Virginia

Mary L. Chavez, PharmD, FAACP
Professor and Chair of Pharmacy Practice
Rangel College of Pharmacy
Texas A&M Health Science Center
Kingsville, Texas

Anisa Fornoff, PharmD
Professor
College of Pharmacy and Health Sciences
Drake University
Des Moines, Iowa

**Benjamin Gross, PharmD, BCPS, BCACP,
    CDE, BC-ADM**
Associate Professor
College of Pharmacy
Lipscomb University
Nashville, Tennessee

Patricia E. Lieveld, PharmD, MPH
Professor
Feik School of Pharmacy
University of the Incarnate Word
San Antonio, Texas

Jodie V. Malhotra, PharmD
International Affairs Coordinator, Distance
    Degrees and Programs
Assistant Professor, Clinical
Skaggs School of Pharmacy and
    Pharmaceutical Sciences
University of Colorado
Denver, Colorado

Jennifer L. Mathews, PhD
Assistant Professor
Wegmans School of Pharmacy
St. John Fisher College
Rochester, New York

Beth Musil, PharmD, CDE
Assistant Professor
School of Pharmacy
Concordia University, Wisconsin
Mequon, Wisconsin

Paul Oesterman, PharmD
Associate Professor
College of Pharmacy
Roseman University of Health Sciences
Henderson, Nevada

Charles D. Ponte, BSc, PharmD, DPNAP, FAPhA, FASHP, FCCP
Professor
School of Pharmacy
West Virginia University
Morgantown, West Virginia

Charles D. Shively, PhD, RPh
Associate Professor
School of Pharmacy
Presbyterian College
Clinton, South Carolina

Angela Thompson, PharmD, BCPS
Assistant Professor
School of Pharmacy
University of Wyoming
Cheyenne, Wyoming

Katy E. Trinkley, PharmD, BCACP
Assistant Professor
Skaggs School of Pharmacy and
  Pharmaceutical Sciences
University of Colorado
Aurora, Colorado

Lucien L. Van Elsen, BS, RPh
Instructor
Milwaukee Area Technical College
Milwaukee, Wisconsin

Bree Watzak, PharmD, BCPS
Assistant Professor
Rangel College of Pharmacy
Texas A&M Health Science Center
Kingsville, Texas

Preparing for the Provision of Culturally Competent Pharmaceutical Care

How Does One Prepare for Culturally Competent Patient Care?

One can apply the statement "preparation is key" to many aspects of life. Preparation can help lead to successful outcomes in the classroom, in one's career, and in one's personal life. For healthcare providers, preparation for providing quality care to patients involves not only learning about clinical presentation of disease and its management, but also learning about a patient's beliefs, values, and culture, and how they can influence the patient's views on illness and management.

Cultural competency and providing culturally competent care is being emphasized more in the healthcare field. Some may wonder, "How does providing *culturally competent patient care* differ from providing *patient care*?" Indeed there is a difference, and this difference can impact the following:

- How the provider asks questions to gather information
- Who the provider speaks with when conducting a patient interview
- The responses the provider may receive from the patient about the medical condition
- What additional information the provider may view as pertinent when assessing the patient
- What is involved in the treatment plan

© entistock/Shutterstock, Inc.

Unit I begins to address the aforementioned items. In addition, the unit includes a discussion on why the provision of culturally competent care in the healthcare arena is important. This discussion includes an overview on health disparities, elements of culture, and cultural competency. Finally, this unit will discuss how pharmacists can become culturally competent patient care providers.

Chapter 1

The Case for Culturally Competent Care in Patient Assessment

Yolanda M. Hardy, PharmD
Charisse Johnson, MS, PharmD
Carmita A. Coleman, PharmD, MAA

LEARNING OBJECTIVES

At the completion of this chapter, the reader should be able to:

1. List factors contributing to health disparities and various initiatives to mitigate their existence.
2. Identify and explain theoretical frameworks of cultural competence.
3. Describe various cultural competence assessment tools.
4. Define culturally competent patient care in terms of pharmacy.
5. Describe areas of the pharmaceutical care process that can be affected by culture.

KEY TERMS

Acculturation

Assimilation

Cultural competence

Cultural humility

Culturally competent patient care

Culturally competent pharmacist patient care

Culture

Health disparities

Health equity

Health literacy

Patient assessment

Pharmaceutical care

Physical assessment

Stereotype

Introduction

The role of the pharmacist has evolved to include services related to the provision of patient care that extends beyond medication dispensing and patient counseling services. In a 2009 survey by Schommer et al., 43% of respondents reported that they were providing patient care services to some degree at their place of employment. Medication therapy management (MTM) services enable the pharmacist to become even more involved in

© antishock/Shutterstock, Inc.

Table 1-1 Examples of MTM Services

Anticoagulation management	Chronic disease state management
Immunizations	Medication review
	Pharmacotherapy consults

patient care (**Table 1-1**), thus providing the pharmacist with the opportunity to make an impact on patient health outcomes. Studies such as the Asheville Project, the Diabetes Ten City Challenge, and Project ImPACT: Hyperlipidemia prove that pharmacists can make a significant impact on patient outcomes when they are a part of the medical team (Bunting, 2008; Fera, 2009; Bluml, 2000) (**Table 1-2**).

The goal for all healthcare providers is to ensure that patients achieve optimal health outcomes; however, not all patients achieve this. Differences in health outcomes or health status between population groups are referred to as healthcare inequalities, or **health disparities** (Smedley, 2003; U.S. Department of Health and Human Services [HHS], 2011; World Health Organization). Health disparities can be observed across different ethnic and cultural groups, genders, ages, socioeconomic statuses, or other social or biological determinants (Institute of Medicine, 2002; Smedley, 2003; SteelFisher, 2004; HHS, 2011) (**Table 1-3**).

A single explanation for the presence of health disparities does not exist because many factors can contribute to the development of health disparities. Pharmacists, as patient care providers, should be aware of how these contributors can impact how patient care is provided. The Institute of Medicine (IOM) landmark publication, "Unequal Treatment: Confronting Racial and Ethnic Disparities in Health Care," (2002) reported contributors to health disparities (Smedley, 2003) (**FIGURE 1-1**).

Health disparities: Differences in disease incidence and/or prevalence among various cultural groups.

Table 1-2 Evidence of Pharmacist Impact on Patient Care Outcomes

Pharmacist Collaborative Services	Impact
Asheville Project	Sustained improvements in blood pressure, LDL, TG, and TC Increase in percentage of patients at blood pressure and LDL goals Reduction in cardiovascular event rate Increase in cardiovascular medication use
Diabetes Ten City Challenge	Reduction in A1C, LDL, and blood pressure Increase in influenza vaccinations, eye exams, and foot exams
Project ImPACT: Hyperlipidemia	Reduction in LDL Increase in HDL High medication compliance rates

LDL = low-density lipoprotein; TG = triglycerides; TC = total cholesterol; HDL = high-density lipoprotein
Data from Bunting BA, Smith BH, Sutherland SE. The Asheville Project: clinical and economic outcomes of a community-based long-term medication therapy management program for hypertension and dyslipidemia. *J Am Pharm Assoc.* 2008; 48:23–31; Fera T, Bluml B, Ellis W. Diabetes ten city challenge: Final economic and clinical results. *J Am Pharm Assoc.* 2009;49:e52–e60; and Bluml BM, McKenney JM, Cziraky MJ. Pharmaceutical care services and results in Project ImPACT: hyperlipidemia. *J Am Pharm Assoc (Wash).* 2000 Mar–Apr;40(2):157–65.

Other factors have also been identified as contributors to healthcare disparities (**Table 1-4**); for example, access to health insurance has been determined to be a contributing factor (SteelFisher, 2004). The IOM determined that minority patients are disproportionately enrolled in lower-cost insurance plans, if enrolled in an insurance plan at all (Smedley, 2003; Phillips, 2000). These plans tend to place a greater emphasis on cost containments and healthcare expenditures. This has the potential to affect not only access to quality care, but also access to medication for management of disease. Another contributor to health disparities can result from not asking the patient about his or her preferences in regard to healthcare management and treatment. This can result in providers overlooking preferred treatment options, and thus patient nonadherence to treatment recommendations (Smedley, 2003).

Table 1-3 Examples of Health Disparities in U.S. Populations: Healthy People 2020 Findings

Diabetes prevalence rates among American Indians are 2 to 5 times higher than for their white counterparts.

More than 50% of cases of human immunodeficiency virus (HIV) occur in gay or bisexual men, and 45% of newly diagnosed cases occur in African Americans.

African American women are particularly at risk for infertility issues.

Data from Healthy People 2020: Topics and Objectives. U.S. Department of Health and Human Services. http://www.healthypeople.gov/2020/topicsobjectives2020/default.aspx. Accessed July 26, 2014.

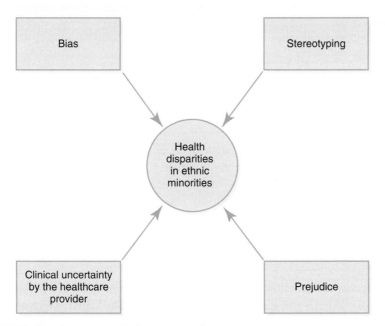

FIGURE 1-1 Contributors to health disparities in ethnic minorities.

Data from Smedley BD, Stith AY, Nelson AR (eds.). Committee on Understanding and Eliminating Racial and Ethnic Disparities in Health Care. *Unequal Treatment: Confronting Racial and Ethnic Disparities in Health Care.* Washington, DC: The National Academies Press; 2003.

Table 1-4 Examples of Contributing Factors to Health Disparities

Income	Access to Care	Differences in Medical Needs
Socioeconomic status	Insurance Access to transportation Number of healthcare facilities and providers available	Patient preferences Differences in severity of illnesses
Differences in Healthcare Delivery	**Language and Cultural Barriers**	**Provider–Patient Interactions**
Fragmentation of healthcare services Provider incentives for cost containment	Language discordance Access to interpretive services Health-seeking behaviors Cultural incongruences	Acceptance of provider recommendations Biases, prejudices, and/or stereotypes Clinical uncertainty Patient mistrust or refusal

Data from Betancourt J, Green A, Carrilo JE. *Cultural Competence in Health Care: Emerging Frameworks and Practical Approaches.* The Commonwealth Fund, October 2002; Smedley BD, Stith AY, Nelson AR (eds.). Committee on Understanding and Eliminating Racial and Ethnic Disparities in Health Care. *Unequal Treatment: Confronting Racial and Ethnic Disparities in Health Care.* Washington, DC: The National Academies Press; 2003; SteelFisher G. *Addressing Unequal Treatment: Disparities in Health Care.* The Commonwealth Fund; November 2004; and Sullivan Commission. *Missing persons: minorities in the health professions: a report of the Sullivan Commission on diversity in the healthcare workforce.* Washington, DC. 2004. Available at http://www.aacn.nche.edu/media-relations/SullivanReport .pdf. Accessed July 18, 2013. Adapted from sources: Betancourt; Smedley; SteelFisher; and Sullivan Commission.

Example

It has been documented that pharmacies in minority or low-income neighborhoods stock fewer narcotic and anxiolytic agents in an effort to thwart theft and burglary. How could this practice contribute to a disparity in health care for patients who reside in these communities?

Health equity: Attainment of the highest level of health for all people (HHS, 2011).

A concerted effort has been made to eliminate health disparities and achieve health equity. This effort is multifaceted, targeting many areas of the healthcare system as well as governmental agencies, educational systems, professional organizations, and the healthcare industry. Federal and legislative initiatives, such as the National Standards on Culturally and Linguistically Appropriate Services (CLAS), have helped address some of the factors that contribute to health disparities. CLAS help to ensure that healthcare organizations make healthcare and related services more accessible by offering language assistance services to patients (HHS, 2014). Healthy People 2010, spearheaded by the U.S. Department of Health and Human Services, was developed in 2000 with the primary goals of eliminating health disparities and increasing the quantity and quality of healthy life years nationwide. The Healthy People initiative has continued with the release of Healthy People 2020.

In response to the Sullivan Commission (2004) recommendation for cross-cultural education of healthcare providers, health professions schools, including colleges and schools of pharmacy, have initiated programs and curricula to impact health disparities and promote cross-cultural education (Accreditation Council for Pharmacy Education [ACPE], 2011; Association of American Medical Colleges, 2005; American Association of Colleges of

Nursing, 2008). Implementation of cross-cultural education can help to develop health-care providers who are culturally aware and able to incorporate cultural elements into their patient care practices. The ACPE (2011) standards and guidelines for the professional program in pharmacy leading to the doctor of pharmacy degree now require that "the college or school must ensure that the curriculum addresses patient safety, cultural competence, health literacy, healthcare disparities, and competencies needed to work as a member of or on an interprofessional team" (p. 18). As a result, colleges and schools of pharmacy have incorporated coursework and clinical practice experiences that will help prepare student pharmacists to address health disparities in their careers. Leading pharmacy organizations have also responded to the call to action in regard to eliminating health disparities (ASHP, 2008; American Pharmacists Association, 2013; Vanderpool, 2005). One of the nation's professional pharmacy organizations, the American Society of Health-Systems Pharmacists (ASHP), developed rationale for the culturally appropriate provision of pharmacy services, stating that pharmacists are positioned to be leaders in this arena.

Pharmacists should be viewed as an effective member of the healthcare team dedicated to eliminating healthcare disparities. Pharmacists have shown that their efforts can make a significant impact on patient care outcomes. Coupled with the curricular changes in pharmacy education as well as the positions taken by influential pharmacy organizations, it is clear that pharmacists are in a key position to help eliminate health disparities and thus achieve health equity. Consequently, it is important for pharmacists to understand and utilize models of **culturally competent patient care**, which has been defined by Betancourt, et al. (2002) as "providing care to patients with diverse values, beliefs, and behaviors, including tailoring delivery to meet patients' social, cultural, and linguistic needs." In order to provide such patient care, one must have an understanding of the concepts related to culture, and how these concepts can be applied to health care and, in particular, pharmacy practice.

Beginning the Journey of Providing Culturally Competent Patient Care

To begin the journey toward providing culturally competent patient care, the pharmacist should first realize that **culture** is not just limited to race and ethnicity. This term encompasses language, values, beliefs, behaviors, and traditions. Cultural identity can be based on a multitude of factors, such as age, gender, area of residence, or religion (Johnson, 2005; Kronish, 2012; Coronado, 2004; Patcher, 1994). Culture can influence a person's beliefs and actions in regard to when to seek medical treatment, who to seek treatment from, and how medical conditions are viewed and treated. It is important to keep in mind that not all cultural beliefs, values, traditions, or practices are exactly the same for each patient of a particular culture. This is the result of the processes referred to as acculturation and assimilation.

Acculturation is a process in which an individual begins to incorporate some of the beliefs, values, and traditions of other cultures into his or her life. As a result, one must be aware that not all members of a culture will strictly follow the values, beliefs, traditions, and practices endemic to that culture. In some instances people may experience **assimilation** to the primary or mainstream dominant culture; therefore, cultural practices may not be totally reflective of one specific cultural group. It is important to realize that although

Culturally competent patient care: Care that takes into account social, linguistic, and other individual aspects of the patient.

Culture: The values, attitudes, beliefs, norms, traditions, language, and so on that are characteristic to a group.

Acculturation: To adopt or borrow cultural traits or social patterns from another group.

Assimilation: The process in which an individual or members of a culture come to resemble those of another culture. Full assimilation occurs when new members of the group are indistinguishable from other members of the group.

Stereotype:
A broad generalization, positive or negative, that is associated with a specific group of people.

cultures are unique and vary significantly with respect to values, beliefs, and practices, individuals within the culture are just as unique. Failure of healthcare providers to take this into consideration may allow them to perceive patients as **stereotypes** based on what may be known about some patients' identified ethnic cultural group. Clinical decision making based largely on stereotypes without further inquiry about the individual patient's needs may be detrimental to the pharmacist-patient relationship. Providing patient care based on stereotypes, however, is distinctly different from providing patient care that involves making *informed* decisions rooted in cultural knowledge. For example, it would be important to address known risk factors present in patients of a particular cultural group if those risk factors could potentially lead to poor patient outcomes. Incorporation of this knowledge into one's practice is one of the key elements of reducing health disparities.

Health Literacy

Health literacy:
The ability of an individual to utilize health-related information to make decisions about their own health and health-related issues.

The U.S. Department of Health and Human Services (2000) defines **health literacy** as "the degree to which an individual has the capacity to obtain, communicate, process, and understand basic health information and services to make appropriate health decisions." At least four sections of the law directly reference interventions to impact health literacy, and another six sections may indirectly affect it (Somers, 2010). Statistically, it has been estimated that 87 million adults in the United States are functionally illiterate, which means they have difficulty with the basic understanding and use of written information. More specifically, only about 12% of American adults have a proficient level of health literacy (Somers, 2010). Health literacy is not just a matter of a patient being able to read or write. A patient needs to be able to read, write, speak, listen, perform mathematical calculations, and understand rhetoric or contextual hints to successfully navigate the healthcare system. Unfortunately, many patients are unable to amalgamate these skills appropriately to receive care. It has been estimated that 9 out of 10 adults are not fully able to use health information that is readily available in healthcare facilities and from providers, as well as the health information in everyday media (HHS, 2010).

Low health literacy can adversely impact different types of people, but it has been shown to disproportionately impact nonwhite ethnicities (including minorities), geriatric patients, those with lower socioeconomic status or education, cognitively impaired patients, non-native English speakers, and/or those with low English proficiency (HHS, 2010). These are similar to populations that have previously been identified as being at risk for health disparities. Therefore, a discussion of health literacy must occur in the course of providing culturally competent care. Cultural or linguistic barriers may be inadvertently placed, prohibiting optimal **patient assessment** and care activities.

Patient assessment:
Process used to identify patient problems via evaluation of the patient's subjective reports and objective data.

Health literacy is composed of both individual and systemic factors (**FIGURE 1-2**). Each of those factors contributes to the success of the patient being able to access, receive, and utilize services in the healthcare system. The Centers for Disease Control and Prevention (CDC) has listed the individual factors as literacy skills, health knowledge, demographics/culture, and experience. Each of these determinants is unique to each patient. Systemically, contributory factors are the type of health practice available, the infrastructure of services, and the abilities of the practitioners available to the patient. Practitioners are responsible for the manner of communication and reinforcement that they provide. Increasing the

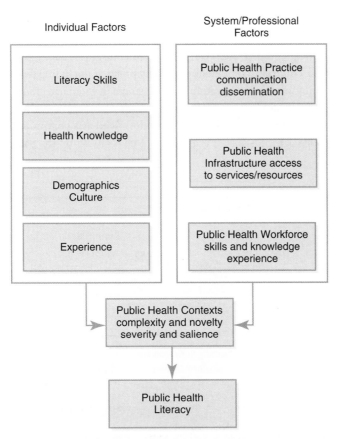

Individual Factors

System/Professional Factors

Literacy Skills

Health Knowledge

Demographics Culture

Experience

Public Health Practice communication dissemination

Public Health Infrastructure access to services/resources

Public Health Workforce skills and knowledge experience

Public Health Contexts complexity and novelty severity and salience

Public Health Literacy

FIGURE 1-2 Factors that affect health literacy.

Reproduced from the Centers for Disease Control and Prevention. Health literacy for public health professionals. Available at: http://www.cdc.gov/healthliteracy/training/page655.html. Accessed March 4, 2014.

ease of entry into the healthcare system using simplified forms, unambiguous language, and adequate examples, and probing for understanding are required for the low health literacy patient. Although this brief overview will not review the application of readability scales to patient literature to determine its complexity, the practitioner who is continuously aware that low health literacy is a prevalent issue will interact with a more satisfied, responsive patient. When attempting to develop a successful treatment plan during patient assessment, the practitioner is able to collect more valuable information from a patient who is comfortable and responsive.

Cultural Competence: Definition and Theoretical Frameworks

Recognizing cultural differences is just one part of becoming a culturally competent provider. However, what exactly does it mean to become "culturally competent"? Cross et al. (1989) have defined **cultural competence** as "a set of congruent behaviors, attitudes, and policies that come together in a system, agency or among professionals and enable that system, agency or those professions to work effectively in cross-cultural situations."

Cultural competence: The ability to provide care that takes into account social, linguistic, and other individual aspects of the patient.

Cross's definition of cultural competence underscores a multilayered approach involving not only individuals, but also the policies, procedures, and systems of an organization that are symbiotically intertwined. O'Connell and colleagues (2009) described several components of a "culturally competent pharmacy practice" including developing strong ties with the community and the continuous assessment of whether a practice is achieving culturally competent care.

The cultural competence process has been described as a continuum that consists of six stages (**Table 1-5**). Because it is a process, one is always on the path to becoming

Table 1-5 Stages of Cultural Competence

Stage	Definition	Example
Cultural destructiveness	The presence of practices that are harmful to a cultural group	A practitioner may openly discriminate against an individual or a group of individuals of a specific cultural group by refusing to provide care or services (e.g., a pharmacist refuses to offer interpreter or translator services).
Cultural incapacity	Having the inability to respond to the needs, preferences, or practices of culturally diverse groups; may be the result of a lack of resources, cultural bias, or lower expectations of cultures	It is cost prohibitive for a pharmacist/pharmacy to provide and offer interpreter or translator services to ESL (English as a second language) patients.
Cultural blindness	Stems from the belief of treating all people the same; may encourage assimilation rather than recognizing differences	Pharmacy/pharmacist provides patient education to an ESL patient population only in English and doesn't understand the importance of offering interpreter or translator services.
Cultural precompetence	Having an awareness of areas of strength related to culture and areas of needed improvement; has made efforts to incorporate culture into practice	Pharmacy/pharmacist purchases software that enables the staff to provide patient education in other languages.
Cultural competence	Cultural awareness and practices are implemented into the practice structure	Pharmacy/pharmacist provides an array of interpreter or translator services such as hiring bilingual staff.
Cultural proficiency	Integrates culture into the foundation of all practices and decisions	Pharmacy/pharmacist provides an array of interpreter or translator services and continually assesses the effectiveness and impact of services on patient health outcomes and satisfaction.

Data from Cross T, Bazron B, Dennis K, Isaacs M. *Towards a Culturally Competent System of Care*. Vol. I. Washington, DC: Georgetown University Child Development Center, CASSP Technical Assistance Center; 1989.

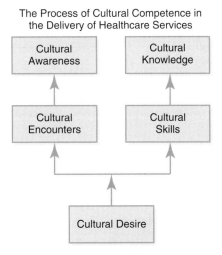

The Process of Cultural Competence in
the Delivery of Healthcare Services

FIGURE 1-3 The process of cultural competence in the delivery of healthcare services.

Reproduced from Campinha-Bacote J. The process of cultural competence in the delivery of healthcare services: A model of care. *J Transcult Nurs.* 2002;13:181.

culturally competent and should be cautioned against the belief that one can develop total mastery of cultural competence.

Additionally, in the article "The Process of Cultural Competence in the Delivery of Healthcare Services: A Model of Care," Campinha-Bacote (2002) conveys that cultural competence is composed of a number of constructs, principally "cultural desire," "cultural awareness," "cultural knowledge," "cultural skills," and "cultural encounters" (**FIGURE 1-3**). According to Campinha-Bacote, a healthcare professional on the pathway to becoming culturally competent regularly self-assesses for individual biases and prejudices (*cultural awareness*), possesses the motivation (*cultural desire*) to continually seek relevant knowledge about various cultural groups (*cultural knowledge*), applies that information appropriately in the provision of direct patient care services (*cultural assessment*), and seeks out experiences (*cultural encounters*) that allow the individual to hone his or her skills. Tervalon and Murray-Garcia (2009) particularly underscored the criticality of self-assessing and reflecting on an individual's cultural identity and the dynamic interplay when interacting with patients as healthcare providers strive for "cultural humility."

> **Cultural humility:** An individual's process of self-introspection and reflection in the quest to respect the diverse values, attitudes, beliefs, norms, and traditions of others.

Cultural Competence Assessment Tools

When beginning the journey toward providing culturally competent patient care, it is a good idea to determine the baseline level of cultural competence. A number of assessment tools (**Table 1-6**) have been published to help individuals measure their ability to provide culturally competent care. Given that becoming able to provide culturally competent care is a process involving motivation, introspection, and the attainment of knowledge and skills, assessment is a vital component of this process.

Table 1-6 Cultural Competency Self-Assessment Tools

Competence Assessment Tool	Method	Cost	Tool Location
Inventory for Assessing the Process of Cultural Competence Among Healthcare Professionals-Revised (IAPCC-R)	Paper-based self-assessment	User fee required	http://www.transculturalcare.net/iapcc-r.htm
Clinical Cultural Competency Questionnaire (CCCQ)	Available online (with explicit author permission)	Free	http://rwjms.rutgers.edu/departments_institutes/family_medicine/chfcd/grants_projects/aetna.html
Cultural Competence Health Practitioner Assessment (CCHPA)	Paper-based self-assessment (with explicit author permission)	Free	http://nccc.georgetown.edu/features/CCHPA.html
Quality and Culture Quiz	Available online	Free	http://erc.msh.org/mainpage.cfm?file=3.0.htm&module=provider

Inventory for Assessing the Process of Cultural Competence Among Healthcare Professionals-Revised

The Inventory for Assessing the Process of Cultural Competence Among Healthcare Professionals-Revised (IAPCC-R), developed in 2002 by Campinha-Bacote, measures the ability of both practitioners and students in medicine and allied health sciences to provide culturally competent care (Transcultural Care Associates, 2002). Administered as a paper-based self-assessment, the IAPCC-R consists of 25 items measuring the cultural competency constructs of desire, awareness, knowledge, skill, and encounters. The estimated completion time is approximately 15 minutes. It utilizes Likert scales to measure responses to the items. The inventory requires author permission and submission of a user fee.

Clinical Cultural Competency Questionnaire

The Clinical Cultural Competency Questionnaire (CCCQ) is a self-assessment tool developed by the Center for Healthy Families and Cultural Diversity, Department of Family Medicine, UMDNJ-Robert Wood Johnson Medical School. The CCCQ was initially developed to specifically measure knowledge, skills, comfort level of encounters/situations, and attitudes of physicians providing care to diverse patient populations in conjunction with a cultural competency training program. The CCCQ is a free tool that can be used with explicit permission of the authors. It is a paper-based self-assessment consisting of approximately 75 items.

The CCCQ, with modifications, may be useful to both pharmacy students and pharmacists. For example, Okoro and colleagues (2012) specifically altered the CCCQ to measure the level of clinical cultural competency and health disparities knowledge in third-year PharmD students; consequently, information gathered from the CCCQ also revealed curricular insight as it related to cultural competency content.

Cultural Competence Health Practitioner Assessment

The Cultural Competence Health Practitioner Assessment (CCHPA) was developed by the National Center for Cultural Competence at Georgetown University and is an exclusively online self-assessment tool with the purpose of enhancing the delivery of services to culturally and linguistically diverse communities. The CCHPA completion time is about 20 minutes, and it addresses the constructs of values and belief systems, cultural aspects of epidemiology, clinical decision making, life cycle events, cross-cultural communication, and empowerment/health management. Depending on the responses, results of the CCHPA will characterize "awareness," "knowledge," or "skill" level for each construct. Participants are also provided with a listing of resources (such as web-based journals, textbooks, etc.) to help support ongoing development in those areas.

The CCHPA may be particularly useful for practitioners who want to assess their provision of culturally competent care to a specific ethnic or cultural group. If participants want to assess multiple groups, the CCHPA should be completed for each individual group. The CCHPA is available at no cost to the participant.

Quality and Culture Quiz

The Providers Guide to Quality and Culture, a joint project of the Management Sciences for Health (MSH) and various agencies of the U.S. Department of Health and Human Services can be utilized by both students and practitioners to obtain information on cultural competency and health disparities. Specifically, the Quality and Culture Quiz contains 23 multiple choice and true/false questions that explore content related to topics such as common beliefs/cultural practices, patient adherence, prejudices, and working with an interpreter.

The Quality and Culture Quiz, available online and at no cost to the participant, can be self-administered both online and via a paper-based format. After completion of the quiz, the answers are provided to the participants with a detailed explanation that includes relevant background information to support the correct answer. A high correct score doesn't necessarily denote mastery, but scores should be used to identify areas of strength and those needing improvement in the continuum of an individual's ability to provide culturally competent care. The Quality and Culture Quiz may be useful for pharmacy students and pharmacists alike.

Use of the cultural competence assessment tools such as those listed here provide a starting step toward incorporating cultural competency into the pharmacist practice. These tools will help to serve as a guide for the pharmacist in determining areas related to cultural awareness, knowledge, and skills that are on target and those that need improvement. Pharmacists can reassess their level of cultural competence using these tools as they move toward becoming more culturally competent.

Culturally Competent Pharmacist Patient Care

A definition for culturally competent pharmacist patient care can be developed by merging the definitions for cultural competence by Betancourt (2002) and **pharmaceutical care** defined by the American Society of Health Systems Pharmacists (2003) from an adaptation

Pharmaceutical care: The provision of care that optimizes health outcomes primarily through the use of pharmacotherapeutic agents.

Culturally competent pharmacist patient care:
The ability to provide appropriate pharmacotherapy treatment that takes into account social, linguistic, and other individual aspects of the patient.

Physical assessment:
Examination of the body from head to toe using observation, palpation, percussion, and auscultation.

of the definition from Hepler and Strand (1990), as "the direct, responsible provision of medication-related care for the purpose of achieving definite outcomes that improve a patient's quality of life." Thus, **culturally competent pharmacist patient care** can be described as the direct, responsible provision of medication-related care to patients with diverse values, beliefs, and behaviors, including tailoring delivery to meet patients' social, cultural and linguistic needs, for the purpose of achieving definite outcomes that improve a patient's quality of life. The remainder of the chapter will provide an overview of how culture can be incorporated into each step of the patient care process.

Information Gathering

Gathering patient-related information is one of the beginning steps in the pharmaceutical care process. Gathering information can be achieved by reviewing the patient's chart, interviewing the patient, and performing **physical assessments**. These steps can allow the pharmacist to better identify the presence or absence of drug-related problems and assess drug therapy outcomes.

Viewing the patient's chart will provide the clinician with not only demographic information, but also information regarding current and past medical conditions, medication history, response to therapies, and patient needs. During the patient interview, sources of information about the patient will include the patient and/or the patient's caregivers and loved ones. The pharmacist will be able to obtain subjective information regarding the patient's current disease state, self-care management of the disease state, and medication adherence and medication-related problems. Performing a physical assessment will provide the pharmacist with the opportunity to gather objective patient data. These data are helpful in determining the extent of disease state control, response to treatment, and the presence of drug-related problems.

Cultural Considerations: Information Gathering

During the information gathering process, finding cultural information in the patient's chart can be valuable. The patient's chart can provide some insight regarding the patient's anticipated needs, such as communication needs, the language preferred to be spoken when discussing healthcare issues, and the patient's race and ethnicity. Some charts may also include information about the patient's gender, sexual identity, or religious practices, which could be helpful when formulating a care plan for the patient. Information such as the patient's communication needs, race, and ethnicity is now required to be in patient charts by some accrediting bodies (The Joint Commission, 2010). Knowing the patient's communication needs in advance of the patient visit and addressing those needs will allow more information gathering during the patient interview and will reduce the chances of communication errors, which could lead to drug-related errors (Divi, 2007). Being aware of the patient's race and ethnicity prior to the visit will aid in making informed decisions about how to address risk factors and/or health disparities reported in those particular groups. With this information, the pharmacist can create a patient-specific care plan that addresses the patient's needs.

Certainly addressing the language needs of the patient will be imperative for the patient interview; however, other cultural considerations also should be noted during the interview process. In addition to language differences, cultural nuances related to the use of verbal and nonverbal communication can affect how information sought or provided is interpreted by either party. Cultural beliefs regarding who makes health-related decisions may affect who is responding to the information-gathering questions (Institute for Safe Medication Practices, 2003; EuroMed Info; Blackhall, 1995). Finally, cultural views on disease development, health-seeking practices, and origins of illness may be misinterpreted or unintentionally ignored, thus again affecting the patient–pharmacist relationship and ultimately treatment outcomes. To help overcome this, the pharmacist may need to utilize a different series of open-ended questions to gather more information for a better understanding.

Although the physical assessment performed by the pharmacist is pretty limited compared to what is performed by other healthcare professionals, awareness of the cultural implications is still important. In some cultures modesty is highly regarded, which may result in requests for examinations being performed by providers of the same gender (Carteret, 2011).

Identification of Drug-Related Problems

Findings from the information-gathering step of the process should aid in the evaluation for the presence or absence of a drug-related problem (DRP). DRPs have been classified into the categories shown in **Table 1-7**.

Table 1-7 Drug-Related Problems

Untreated indication	Improper drug selection
Subtherapeutic dose	Failure to receive medication
Supratherapeutic dose	Adverse drug reaction
Drug interaction	Medication use without indication

Data from American Society of Hospital Pharmacists. ASHP statement on pharmaceutical care. *Am J Hosp Pharm.* 1993; 50:1720–3; Hepler CD, Strand LM. Opportunities and responsibilities in pharmaceutical care. *Am J Hosp Pharm.* 1990; 47:533–543.

Cultural Considerations: Identification of a Drug-Related Problem

Culture plays a role in the identification of a drug-related problem as well as the reason for the drug-related problem. As an example, an untreated indication may be due to the patient not believing that the condition needs to be treated with medication, and as a result, the patient chooses to not take the prescribed medication. The decision to use an herbal product rather than the medication prescribed by the physician may result in the drug-related problem of a subtherapeutic dose if the patient didn't tell the healthcare provider that they were using herbal products rather than taking the prescription drug. In this case, the provider may have created a plan that consisted of continuous dose escalations and possibly the addition of more medications.

Formulating a Plan

The medication-related aspects of developing a pharmaceutical care plan involve evaluating the need for medication therapy and developing a safe, appropriate, and effective medication plan for a patient. It also includes the provision of medication education to the patient in the form of patient counseling and establishing an appropriate follow-up and monitoring plan to ensure efficacy of the plan.

Cultural Considerations: Formulating a Plan

Creating a drug therapy plan and execution of the plan can be impacted by culture. Although the focus of this text is not on drug selection based on cultural pharmacogenomic variances, it is important to note that drug selection may be guided by cultural or ethnic differences. The creation and execution of the plan can be impacted in other ways. A patient's cultural or spiritual beliefs can impact whether a patient believes he or she needs medication for a certain illness, which can affect adherence to medications (Kretchy, 2013). If the pharmacist believes that the patient needs a medication, yet the patient does not, it may lead to a cultural impasse that can hinder the ability to achieve effective patient outcomes. These are just a few examples of what should be considered when creating and executing the drug therapy plan; failure to address these issues, and those that are similar, can affect patient outcomes.

Summary

This chapter has highlighted the need to provide culturally competent care as one strategy to mitigate health disparities. The relationship between culture and the pharmaceutical care process was explored in terms of how pharmacists can specifically provide culturally competent pharmacist patient care, because culture can have an impact on each step of the process. Additionally, the theoretical frameworks and assessment tools provide the reader with guidance to assist in the overall development of becoming a culturally competent provider.

As a member of the healthcare team, pharmacists have a responsibility to provide care to patients that is designed to ensure positive outcomes for all patients. Incorporating the patient's cultural beliefs and needs is key in this process.

Review Questions

1. In "The Process of Cultural Competence in the Delivery of Healthcare Services: A Model of Care," Campinha-Bacote describes that cultural competence is composed of a number of constructs. What actions and/or behaviors would an individual display in the "cultural desire" construct?

2. YL is a 50-year-old man who presents to the pharmacy with a prescription for lisinopril, an antihypertensive agent. You look in YL's profile and see that he was prescribed this medication 6 months ago, and again 2 months ago, but he never picked up the medication. Today you notice that the medication dose has been increased. YL speaks very little English, and you do not speak French, which is his preferred language, as listed in his profile. Via an interpreter, you learn that YL stopped taking the lisinopril after 1 week of taking it because he "felt that he didn't have high blood pressure anymore." He did not tell the doctor this because he did not want to disrespect him. Using the interpreter, you were able to speak to YL more about hypertension and treatment. You also inquired more about his beliefs, and what he thought about treating his hypertension. In the end, YL agreed to take the antihypertensive medication. You then called

the physician, explained your findings, and suggested that the lisinopril dose be reduced to a lower dose.

Explain how culture influenced each part of the patient care process in this scenario.

3. JP, a 46-year-old woman, arrives to the clinic for a glucometer teaching and medication review. Prior to starting the visit, what types of information would you look for in her chart to help plan for a culturally competent patient visit? Explain your rationale for your answer.

4. JP returns to the clinic 2 weeks later with a blood glucose log. You see that her blood sugars have been really low. You are concerned about hypoglycemia, and therefore you recommend to her physician to reduce her insulin dose. The physician agrees, and reduces the dose. While explaining to JP the new dose, she explains to you that she is participating in a 21-day fast with her church, in which she has had to eliminate meats and bread from her diet; she eats only fruits and vegetables, and drinks water. How would the patient care process have been affected had JP not shared the information regarding the fast with you? Why?

References

Accreditation Council for Pharmacy Education (ACPE). Accreditation standards and guidelines for the professional program in pharmacy leading to the doctor of pharmacy degree. Available at: http://www.acpe-accredit.org/pdf/FinalS2007Guidelines2.0.pdf. Published January 23, 2011. Accessed March 30, 2013.

American Association of Colleges of Nursing. Cultural competency in baccalaureate nursing education. Available at: http://www.aacn.nche.edu/leading-initiatives/education-resources/competency.pdf. Accessed August 14, 2014.

American Pharmacists Association. APhA policy disparities in health care. *JAPhA*. 2009;NS49(4):493. Available at: http://www.pharmacist.com/policy/disparities-health-care-15. Accessed August 15, 2014.

American Pharmacists Association. What is medication therapy management? APhA MTM Central. Available at: http://www.pharmacist.com/mtm. Accessed July 18, 2013.

American Society of Health-System Pharmacists. ASHP statement on racial and ethnic disparities in health care. *Am J Health Syst Pharm*. 2008;65:728–733.

American Society of Hospital Pharmacists. ASHP statement on pharmaceutical care. *Am J Hosp Pharm*. 1993;50:1720–1723.

Association of American Medical Colleges. Cultural competence education. Available at: https://www.aamc.org/download/54338/data/culturalcomped.pdf. Published 2005. Accessed August 15, 2014.

Betancourt J, Green A, Carrilo JE. *Cultural Competence in Health Care: Emerging Frameworks and Practical Approaches*. The Commonwealth Fund; October 2002.

Blackhall L, Murphy S, Frank G, Michel V, Azen S. Ethnicity and attitudes toward patient autonomy. *JAMA*. 1995;274(10):821–825.

Bluml BM, McKenney JM, Cziraky MJ. Pharmaceutical care services and results in project ImPACT: hyperlipidemia. *J Am Pharm Assoc (Wash)*. 2000;40(2):157–165.

Bunting BA, Smith BH, Sutherland SE. The Asheville Project: clinical and economic outcomes of a community-based long-term medication therapy management program for hypertension and dyslipidemia. *J Am Pharm Assoc.* 2008;48:23–31.

Campinha-Bacote J. The process of cultural competence in the delivery of healthcare services: a model of care. *J Transcult Nurs.* 2002;13:181–184.

Carteret M. Modesty in health care: a cross-cultural perspective. Dimensions of Culture: Cross-Cultural Communications for Health Care Professionals. 2011. Available at: http://www.dimensionsofculture.com/2010/11/modesty-in-health-care-a-cross-cultural-perspective. Accessed July 18, 2013.

Centers for Disease Control and Prevention. Health literacy for public health professionals. Available at: http://www.cdc.gov/healthliteracy/training/page655.html. Accessed March 4, 2014.

Centers for Disease Control and Prevention. Learn about health literacy. Available at: http://www.cdc.gov/healthliteracy/learn/index.html. Accessed March 3, 2014.

Commission on Social Determinants of Health. *Closing the Gap in a Generation: Health Equity Through Action on the Social Determinants of Health.* Geneva: World Health Organization; 2008. Available at: http://whqlibdoc.who.int/publications/2008/9789241563703_eng.pdf. Accessed July 18, 2013.

Coronado G, Thompson B, Tejeda S, Godina R. Attitudes and beliefs among Mexican Americans about type 2 diabetes. J Health Care Poor Underserved. 2004;15(4):576–588.

Cross T, Bazron B, Dennis K, Isaacs M. *Towards a Culturally Competent System of Care.* Vol. I. Washington, DC: Georgetown University Child Development Center, CASSP Technical Assistance Center; 1989.

Divi C, Koss R, Schmaltz S, Loeb J. Language proficiency and adverse events in US hospitals: a pilot study. *Int J Qual Health Care.* 2007;19:60–67.

EuroMed Info. How culture influences health beliefs. Available at: http://www.euromedinfo.eu/how-culture-influences-health-beliefs.html. Accessed August 16, 2014.

Fera T, Bluml B, Ellis W. Diabetes ten city challenge: final economic and clinical results. *J Am Pharm Assoc.* 2009;49:e52–e60.

Hepler CD, Strand LM. Opportunities and responsibilities in pharmaceutical care. *Am J Hosp Pharm.* 1990;47:533–543.

Institute for Safe Medication Practices. Cultural diversity and medication safety. 2003. Available at: http://www.ismp.org/newsletters/acutecare/articles/20030904.asp. Accessed July 18, 2013.

Institute of Medicine. Unequal treatment: what healthcare providers need to know about racial and ethnic disparities in healthcare. 2002. Available at: http://www.iom.edu/~/media/Files/Report%20Files/2003/Unequal-Treatment-Confronting-Racial-and-Ethnic-Disparities-in-Health-Care/Disparitieshcproviders8pgFINAL.pdf. Accessed July 18, 2013.

Johnson KS, Elbert-Avila KI, Tulsky JA. The influence of spiritual beliefs and practices on the treatment preferences of African Americans: a review of the literature. *J Am Geriatr Soc.* 2005;53:711–719.

Kretchy I, Owusu-Daaku F, Danquah S. Spiritual and religious beliefs: do they matter in the medication adherence behaviour of hypertensive patients? *BioPsychoSocial Medicine.* 2013;7(15):1–7.

Kronish I, Leventhal H, Horowitz C. Understanding minority patients' beliefs about hypertension to reduce gaps in communication between patients and clinicians. *J Clin Hypertens.* 2012;14(1):38–44.

Like RC. Clinical cultural competency questionnaire (pre-training version). Center for Healthy Families and Cultural Diversity, Department of Family Medicine, UMDNJ-Robert Wood Johnson Medical School. Available at: http://rwjms.umdnj.edu/departments_institutes/family_medicine/chfcd/grants_projects/documents/Pretraining.pdf. Published 2001. Accessed March 30, 2013.

Management Sciences for Health. The provider's guide to quality and culture. The quality and culture quiz. Available at: http://erc.msh.org/mainpage.cfm?file=3.0.htm&module=provider. Accessed July 18, 2013.

National Center for Cultural Competence, Georgetown University Center for Child and Human Development. Cultural competence health practitioner assessment (CCHPA) overview/purpose. Available at: http://nccc.georgetown.edu/features/CCHPA.html. Accessed July 18, 2013.

National Center for Cultural Competence, Georgetown University Center for Child and Human Development. Curricula enhancement module series: glossary. Available at: http://www.ncccurricula.info/glossary.html. Accessed 8/15/14.

O'Connell MB, Rickles NM, Sias JJ, Korner EJ. Cultural competency in health care and its implications for pharmacy, part 2. Emphasis on pharmacy systems and practice. *Pharmacotherapy.* 2009;29(2):14e–34e.

Okoro ON, Odedina FT, Reams RR, Smith WT. Clinical cultural competency and knowledge of health disparities among pharmacy students. *Am J Pharm Educ.* 2012;76(3):40.

Patcher L. Culture and clinical care: folk illnesses and behaviors and their implications for health care delivery. *JAMA.* 1994;271(9):690–694.

Phillips KA, Mayer ML, Aday LA. Barriers to care among racial ethnic groups under managed care. *Health Aff.* 2000;19(4):65–75.

Rutgers Robert Wood Johnson Medical School, Department of Family Medicine and Community Health, Center for Healthy Families and Cultural Diversity. Cultural competency/quality improvement study. Available at: http://rwjms.rutgers.edu/departments_institutes/family_medicine/chfcd/grants_projects/aetna.html. Accessed July 18, 2013.

Schommer JC, Planas LG, Johnson KA, Doucette WR, Gaither CA, Kreling DH, Mott DA. Pharmacist contributions to the U.S. health care system. *Innovations in Pharmacy.* 2010;1(1) Article 7.

Smedley BD, Stith AY, Nelson AR (eds.). Committee on Understanding and Eliminating Racial and Ethnic Disparities in Health Care. *Unequal Treatment: Confronting Racial and Ethnic Disparities in Health Care.* Washington, DC: The National Academies Press; 2003.

Somers SA, Mahadevan R. Health literacy implications of the Affordable Care Act. Center for Health Care Strategies. Available at: http://www.chcs.org/usr_doc/Health_Literacy_Implcations_of_the_Affordable_Care_Act.pdf. Accessed March 3, 2014.

SteelFisher G. *Addressing Unequal Treatment: Disparities in Health Care.* The Commonwealth Fund; November 2004.

Sullivan Commission. Missing persons: minorities in the health professions: a report of the Sullivan Commission on Diversity in the Healthcare Workforce. 2004. Available at: http://www.aacn.nche.edu/media-relations/SullivanReport.pdf. Accessed July 18, 2013.

Tervalon M, Murray-Garcia J. Cultural humility versus cultural competence: a critical distinction in defining physician training outcomes in multicultural education. *J Health Care Poor Underserved*. 2009; 9:2.

The Joint Commission. *Advancing Effective Communication, Cultural Competence, and Patient- and Family-Centered Care: A Roadmap for Hospitals*. Oakbrook Terrace, IL: The Joint Commission; 2010.

Transcultural CARE Associates. Inventory for assessing the process of cultural competence among health care professionals-revised (IAPCC-R). Available at: http://www.transculturalcare.net/iapcc-r.htm. Published 2002. Accessed July 18, 2013.

U.S. Department of Health and Human Services. 2000. *Healthy People 2010.* Washington, DC: U.S. Government Printing Office. Originally developed for Ratzan SC, Parker RM. 2000. Introduction. In *National Library of Medicine Current Bibliographies in Medicine: Health Literacy*. Selden CR, Zorn M, Ratzan SC, Parker RM, Editors. NLM Pub. No. CBM 2000-1. Bethesda, MD: National Institutes of Health, U.S. Department of Health and Human Services.

U.S. Department of Health and Human Services. 2020 Topics & Objectives: Diabetes. Available at: http://www.healthypeople.gov/2020/topicsobjectives2020/overview.aspx?topicid=8. Accessed August 16, 2014.

U.S. Department of Health and Human Services. 2020 Topics & Objectives: HIV. Available at: http://www.healthypeople.gov/2020/topicsobjectives2020/overview.aspx?topicid=22. Accessed August 16, 2014.

U.S. Department of Health and Human Services. 2020 Topics & Objectives: Maternal, Infant, and Child Health. Available at: http://www.healthypeople.gov/2020/topicsobjectives2020/overview.aspx?topicid=8. Accessed August 16, 2014.

U.S. Department of Health and Human Services. Healthy people 2010: understanding and improving health. Available at: http://www.healthypeople.gov/2010/document/pdf/uih/2010uih.pdf?visit=1. Accessed June 13, 2013.

U.S. Department of Health and Human Services. Healthy people 2020: about healthy people. Available at: http://www.healthypeople.gov/2020/about/default.aspx. Published December 2010. Accessed August 16, 2014.

U.S. Department of Health and Human Services, Office of Disease Prevention and Health Promotion. National action plan to improve health literacy. Available at: http://www.health.gov/communication/hlactionplan/pdf/Health_Literacy_Action_Plan.pdf. Accessed March 3, 2014.

U.S. Department of Health and Human Services, Office of Minority Health. The national CLAS standards. Available at: http://www.minorityhealth.hhs.gov/omh/browse.aspx?lvl=2&lvlid=53. Updated June 19, 2014. Accessed August 16, 2014.

U.S. Department of Health and Human Services, Office of Minority Health, National Partnership for Action to End Health Disparities. Health equity and disparities. Available at: http://minorityhealth.hhs.gov/npa/templates/browse.aspx?lvl=1&lvlid=34. Accessed July 18, 2013.

Vanderpool H. Report of ASHP ad hoc committee on ethnic diversity and cultural competence. *Am J Health Syst Pharm*. 2005;62:1924–1930.

World Health Organization. Health impact assessment glossary of terms used: F-P. Available at: http://www.who.int/hia/about/glos/en/index1.html. Accessed July 18, 2013.

The Culturally Competent Patient Interview and History

Conducting Patient Interviews and Histories

Conducting patient interviews and histories are two very important skills for pharmacists. The information obtained from patient interviews and histories helps pharmacists identify drug-related problems, assess patient outcomes, and ultimately develop a drug therapy treatment plan (American Pharmacists Association [APhA] Pharmaceutical Care Guidelines Advisory Committee, 1995). Additionally, conducting patient interviews and histories can allow the pharmacist and patient to connect, thereby cultivating the pharmacist–patient relationship (APhA Pharmaceutical Care Guidelines Advisory Committee, 1995). Patient interviews and histories are often done together by the pharmacist.

What Role Does Culture Play in a Patient Interview and History?

As mentioned in Unit I, cultural beliefs can influence patient views on health and treatment of disease. As a result, gaining an understanding of the patient's views can help provide explanations regarding why a patient may refuse to take a certain medication or why a patient delayed seeking medical help for an illness. Incorporating questions regarding the patient's beliefs into the patient interview and history could be of benefit in the following ways:

- Allow for more timely treatment of a condition (e.g., knowing that a patient refuses a certain treatment based on their beliefs can prevent a healthcare provider from recommending that treatment as the first option)

© omtishock/Shutterstock, Inc.

- Help the pharmacist tailor a drug therapy plan that incorporates the patient's belief systems
- Provide an opportunity to educate the patient
- Provide an opportunity for the patient to educate the pharmacist

Unit II focuses on how to gather information such as this when conducting patient interviews and histories. Chapter 2 in this unit will focus on how to conduct a patient interview. It will also include a discussion on focused and comprehensive interviews, as well as patient-centered and clinician-centered interviews. Chapter 3 will continue with a discussion on how to conduct a patient history using various explanatory models that have been designed to assist healthcare providers with conducting a culturally competent patient interview and history.

© omtishock/Shutterstock, Inc.

Chapter 2

The Patient Interview
Yolanda M. Hardy, PharmD

LEARNING OBJECTIVES

At the completion of this chapter, the reader should be able to:

1. Discuss the purpose of the patient interview.
2. Explain the two phases of the approach to patient interviewing.
3. Differentiate between comprehensive and focused interviews.
4. Differentiate between clinician-centered and patient-centered interviews.
5. Explain how the use of patient-centered interviewing can assist in providing a culturally competent patient visit.

KEY TERMS

Clinician-centered interview

Comprehensive interview

Focused interview

Patient-centered interview

Introduction

The patient interview is one component of the information-gathering step of the patient care process. Pharmacist-led patient interviews have undergone transition in response to the ever-increasing role of the pharmacist in providing patient care. The interview can now extend beyond gathering information regarding medication use (APhA Pharmaceutical Care Guidelines Advisory Committee, 1995) (Table 2-1). Information obtained from the patient interview, along with information obtained during the physical assessment, will ultimately help the pharmacist develop the drug therapy treatment plan (APhA Pharmaceutical Care Guidelines Advisory Committee, 1995).

This chapter will focus on how to conduct a patient interview; however, it is important to take into consideration that not all patient care interactions require or lend themselves to performing a patient interview. Therefore, the pharmacist should determine if an

Table 2-1 Purposes of Performing Patient Interviews

Obtain medication histories

Assess medication compliance

Determine patient knowledge on medications or disease state management

Develop a patient-specific treatment plan

Identify the presence or absence of drug-related problems

Determine patient views and beliefs on medication use and disease state

Data from American Society of Hospital Pharmacists. ASHP statement on pharmaceutical care. *Am J Hosp Pharm.* 1993; 50:1720–3; APhA Pharmaceutical Care Guidelines Advisory Committee. Principles of Practice for Pharmaceutical Care. American Pharmacists Association. http://www.pharmacist.com/principles-practice-pharmaceutical-care. Published August 1995. Accessed August 16, 2014.

interview is warranted and if interviewing the patient is the most appropriate manner for gathering patient information.

The level of direct contact with patients may vary between practice settings as well as within practice settings. This can, as a result, influence whether a patient interview can occur. As an example, a pharmacist working on an internal medicine floor in the hospital may be responsible for interviewing patients in order to obtain a medication history, to clarify home medication use, or while providing discharge counseling. On the other hand, a pharmacist rounding in the same hospital on a consult service may not need to interview the patient in order to fulfill the responsibilities required. Furthermore, the state of the patient's condition in the inpatient setting may also determine whether a patient interview is warranted or possible. In these circumstances, the pharmacist may rely on progress notes in the patient chart, other healthcare providers, or the patient's family members to gather information.

Although pharmacists in the outpatient setting have greater direct exposure to patients, certain considerations should be taken into account when determining if a patient interview is appropriate. For example, the pharmacist should consider if the practice setting is conducive to interviewing the patient. Concerns such as privacy and confidentiality should be addressed. The patient will be sharing personal information about their disease and medication history, thoughts, and beliefs, so it is important that other patients are not able to hear the information shared (American Society of Health-System Pharmacists, 1997). Time is also a very important factor. Pharmacists who see patients by appointment for the provision of patient care services will have more opportunity to perform a patient interview because a set amount of time has been devoted to the provision of patient care (Griffith, 1998; Herbert, 2006; Blake, 2009). Pharmacists who see patients in a nonscheduled manner (e.g., a patient who stops by the pharmacy to pick up a prescription) may be able to only briefly interview a patient—if at all—depending on whether the patient or the pharmacist has the time. In these situations, an approach that could be used would be to address urgent medical concerns immediately. Nonurgent concerns could be addressed in a more thorough interview by asking the patient to come back at a scheduled time for further interview.

The Approach to the Interview

The approach to the patient interview can be summarized in two phases: the preparation phase and the execution phase. These two phases are equally important because the better

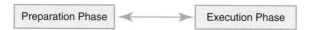

FIGURE 2-1 The relationship between the two phases of the patient interview.

the preparation, the better the pharmacist is able to discover what type of information needs to be gathered during the patient interview. Likewise, the better the execution of the interview, the higher quality and more useful the information received from the patient will be (**FIGURE 2-1**).

Preparation Phase

An effective patient interview begins before the pharmacist even greets the patient; preparation is just as valuable as actually performing the interview. There are three basic steps to follow to assist in preparing for the interview (**FIGURE 2-2**).

Once the pharmacist has determined that an interview is needed, the pharmacist then needs to determine the type of relationship he or she will have with the patient. It is the pharmacist's primary responsibility in all patient relationships to oversee and/or manage drug-related elements of the patient's care; however, other factors come into play when further determining the type of relationship. The pharmacist can further determine the type of relationship by reflecting on the following questions while preparing for the interview (**FIGURE 2-3**). Reflection can help the pharmacist develop questions to ask the patient to assist in gathering information in an efficient manner.

Preparation Phase
• Determine the Relationship • Information Gathering • "Fact Checking"
Execution Phase
• Establish the Relationship • Information Gathering • "Fact Checking"

FIGURE 2-2 Approach to the Patient Interview.

Is this patient new to me?
• A new patient may require a more detailed patient interview. • A returning patient may require a less detailed interview, only focusing on the patient's status since the last encounter.
Why am I seeing this patient today?
• Determining the purpose of the visit can help streamline the information-gathering process.
What is my role in this patient's care?
• Coach? • Educator? • Drug information resource? • Evaluator of drug therapy?

FIGURE 2-3 Reflection questions: Preparing for the interview.

Establishing the Relationship

"Is this patient new to me?"

Comprehensive interview:
An interview style with an encompassing focus that typically involves questioning that addresses all areas of a patient's health history.

Initial visits—the first time the pharmacist is seeing a patient—may warrant a more detailed interview. In this situation, the pharmacist can perform a **comprehensive interview** (Bickley, 2009). Comprehensive interviews are thorough interviews that serve to gather extensive information regarding the patient's history related to medical care. Comprehensive interviews can be extensive; therefore, the pharmacist should take into consideration the practice setting and the urgency of the patient's condition when determining how comprehensive to make the interview. For example, the pharmacist may be able to perform a pretty detailed comprehensive interview for a patient presenting for diabetes management for the first time. However, if the first encounter with a patient is in a more acute setting, such as the emergency room as a result of an adverse drug reaction, it may not be appropriate to perform a detailed, comprehensive interview with the patient. In certain practice settings, such as in the inpatient environment, a comprehensive interview may have already been performed by another healthcare provider on the medical team. In this case, the pharmacist can review the comprehensive interview findings that have been documented in the chart and focus his or her interview on areas that were not addressed, yet are pertinent to the pharmacist's assessment of the patient.

Focused interview:
An interview style with a limited focus that typically involves questioning limited to the patient's chief complaint, a particular disease state, medication use, or the main reason for the patient visit. Often performed during follow-up appointments.

Follow-up visits, in which the pharmacist has seen the patient before for the same medical conditions, do not warrant a comprehensive interview. In this situation, a **focused interview** that consists of gathering new information since the last visit is appropriate (Bickley, 2009). Focused interviews may also be appropriate when the patient is presenting with an acute condition, when the pharmacist is consulted regarding a specific drug-related problem, or when time constraints prevent performing a comprehensive interview.

"Why am I seeing this patient today?"

Having a general idea of the purpose of the patient encounter can help the pharmacist better prepare for the interview (**FIGURE 2-4**). For example, if the purpose of the patient encounter is to provide discharge counseling, then the tasks performed, skills utilized, and questions asked during the encounter will all be related to providing information to the patient about medications that should be used after discharge and ascertaining the patient's level of understanding of the instructions. On the other hand, if the purpose of the encounter is to provide anticoagulation services, then the skills and tasks needed to be performed will focus on evaluating particular lab values, determining the presence or absence of adverse effects and drug interactions, and determining if a new dose is needed.

> **Why Am I Seeing the Patient?**
> • To answer drug information questions
> • To clarify drug dosing
> • For disease state management
> • To identify a drug-related problem
> • For management of a drug-related problem
> • For medication history
> • For medication therapy management
> • For patient education

FIGURE 2-4 Why am I seeing the patient?

"What is my role in the patient's care?"

The pharmacist may serve as a pharmacist care provider, a coach, an educator, or a drug information resource in the patient care process (American Society of Health-System Pharmacists, 1999; Smith et al., 2010; Kaboli P et al., 2006). Each of these roles brings a different level of interaction with the patient as well as different levels of responsibilities for the pharmacist. For example, if a patient has been referred for smoking cessation, the pharmacist's role may be that of a coach in addition to being a pharmacist. In this situation, the pharmacist may celebrate the patient's smoking cessation victories and offer support during periods of difficulty with cravings, all while monitoring drug therapy for efficacy and safety. If the pharmacist is rounding with a medical team in a hospital, his or her role may be as an information resource and educator for the patient, answering questions that the patient or their family may have during the hospital stay and upon discharge, along with monitoring drug therapy while the patient is hospitalized.

Information Gathering

The next step in the preparation phase is information gathering. Being aware of the relationship that the pharmacist will have with the patient can help determine what type of information needs to be gathered during this process. To begin, the pharmacist should review the patient's chart. Reviewing a patient chart for the first time can be a daunting task, especially if time is limited. Familiarizing oneself with the format of the chart can help make the process go by quickly. Another technique that can assist in making a chart review efficient is to have a predetermined list of key information necessary to review for patients who have particular disease states, are taking certain medications, or are of a certain age (**FIGURE 2-5**). Reviewing the patient chart will also help the pharmacist to begin to identify possible drug-related problems. Examples of information that one should be concerned with are listed in **Table 2-2**.

In addition, the pharmacist should review his or her own knowledge base to ensure that he or she is well versed in the patient's disease states and drug therapy regimens.

Example Checklist for Patients with Diabetes
• Medications (insulin vs. oral medication)
• SMBG values
• HA1C
• Renal function
• Height, weight, blood pressure
• Diet and lifestyle
• Complications
• Immunization history
Example Checklist for Patients Taking Statins
• Age
• Lipid panel
• Liver function test
• Drug interactions (grapefruit)
• Muscle soreness, pain
• Headache, dyspepsia
• Concomitant agents that increase risk of myopathy

FIGURE 2-5 Example checklists to assist with reviewing charts.

Table 2-2 Information Gathered from the Patient Chart

Information	Why Is This Important?
Patient name	To help with proper identification of the patient
Age (date of birth)	To help assess if the patient is due for age-related medical screenings To help assess if the patient may need renal dose adjustments
Gender	To help assess if the patient is due for gender-related medical screenings
Preferred language spoken	To determine if an interpreter is needed, thus ensuring that all language needs are met according to culturally and linguistically appropriate services (CLAS) standards
Insurance coverage	To assist in drug therapy decision making by selecting therapeutically effective and cost-effective agents for the patient To help identify the cause of drug-related problems if cost or unavailability on the insurance formulary prevent the patient from purchasing the medication
Employment status/type of employment	To assist in determining drug administration time based on the patient's lifestyle and work schedule To assist in determining helpful lifestyle modification recommendations To help determine affordable medication regimens
Disease state history	To assess for drug-related problems, medication efficacy, and the patient's past response to other agents
Medication list and history	To assess for drug-related problems and the appropriateness of the drug therapy regimen
Drug allergies	To assist in drug therapy selection by omitting agents to which the patient has had a previous allergic reaction
Pertinent lab values	To assess drug therapy outcomes for efficacy and adverse drug events To assess the dose selection of the medication regimen
Pertinent vital signs	To assess drug therapy outcomes for efficacy
Education status	To provide patient education in a manner that is valuable to the patient
Health literacy	To provide patient education in a manner that is valuable to the patient
Adherence	To help determine drug therapy regimens that will improve adherence To assist in determining drug therapy efficacy
Lifestyle (alcohol, tobacco, illicit drug use)	To provide recommendations for risk reduction

Fact Checking

The last step in the preparation process consists of comparing the findings in the chart with the pharmacist's own clinical knowledge base. In essence, this step answers the questions "Does this make sense?" and "What's missing?" This is when the pharmacist can reflect on the following questions:

- Does the drug match the disease state?
- Is the patient on a medication for which there is no indication?
- Is the dose appropriate? Is there room to increase the dose if necessary? Is it renally dosed? Hepatically dosed?
- Are there potential drug–drug interactions?
- Are there potential drug–food interactions?
- Are there potential drug–disease state interactions?
- What side effects should I look for?
- Does the outcome reflect a therapeutic success?
- Based on what I know, are there labs or screening tests that need to be performed?

The aforementioned questions are just an example of what the pharmacist could reflect on during the preparation stage. The questions should be tailored to best fit the purpose of the patient visit. After reviewing the questions, the pharmacist should make note of items that do not make sense or those things that are missing, and inquire about them during the patient interview or during a discussion with the patient's healthcare provider.

Example 1

You are currently a student pharmacist on an internal medicine rotation at a local hospital. You have been assigned to care for a patient who was admitted for community-acquired pneumonia 5 days ago. After reviewing the patient chart, you discover that the patient is on a regimen of antibiotics with an atypical dosing interval. After reviewing the medication administration record for the patient, you question the dosing interval for the antibiotic because it does not make sense. After viewing the patient's labs, you discover that the patient experienced acute renal failure during the early part of his stay in the hospital, and as a result, his antibiotics were renally dosed. The patient's renal function has now returned to normal. As a result, the patient can take the antibiotic at the regular dosing interval. You make note of this information and decide to discuss it with the medical resident during rounds.

Execution Phase

The execution phase begins once the pharmacist has completed all of the steps in the preparation phase and is ready to see the patient. As with the preparation phase, there are three steps to follow during the execution phase: establishing the relationship, information gathering, and fact checking. Success in this phase requires organization and effective use of the time spent with the patient (**FIGURE 2-6**). The pharmacist should be able to accomplish this phase with ease based on the steps taken in the preparation phase.

> **Organization Template for a Patient Visit**
>
> 1) Establishing the Relationship
>   - Introductions
>   - Confirm reason for visit and inquire about patient concerns
> 2) Information Gathering
>   - Gather information by performing patient interview, incorporating open-and closed-ended questions
>   - Gather information by performing physical assessment
> 3) Fact Checking
>   - Answer the questions "Does this make sense?" and "What's missing?"

FIGURE 2-6 Organization template for a patient visit.

Establishing the Relationship

Establishing the relationship with the patient should begin with the pharmacist making an introduction to the patient. Although the role of the pharmacist has expanded and has become accepted by many healthcare professionals, it is important to realize that not all patients have had exposure to pharmacists providing services outside of dispensing medications. As a result, the patient may initially appear a little confused or apprehensive during the start of the visit. Therefore, the pharmacist should introduce him- or herself not only by exchanging names, but also by explaining the reason for the visit. In addition, the pharmacist should inform the patient that the purpose of the visit is also to answer any questions or concerns that he or she may have.

Information Gathering

Once the pharmacist is with the patient, he or she should gather as much information as possible that pertains to the purpose of the visit. The ultimate goal of this step is to address the issues that led to the visit, as well as to identify potential drug-related problems. This step involves both interviewing the patient and performing physical exam techniques.

Often healthcare providers, including pharmacists, start a patient interview with a specific goal in mind, which is to gather the information they need to confirm what they think is wrong with the patient so that they can recommend treatment. Although the clinician gathers valuable information during the interview, this type of interview, referred to as **clinician-centered interviewing**, primarily consists of the clinician asking a series of questions and listening to the patient's response (Fortin et al., 2012). This method of interviewing (**FIGURE 2-7A**) is mostly under the control of the clinician. The clinician typically asks questions to obtain details to help determine the patient's problem based on his or her personal knowledge base (Fortin et al., 2012). In this method of interviewing, the patient's thoughts, perceptions, and concerns about the condition are not considered. The patient may not feel as if the clinician is interested in what they have to say or how they feel. Many clinicians may unintentionally use a clinician-centered approach with a patient, as described in Example 2.

Clinician-centered interview:
An interview style in which the clinician guides the interview in his or her preferred direction. The clinician's issues of concern may be given priority over the patient's concerns. Patient interaction may be limited.

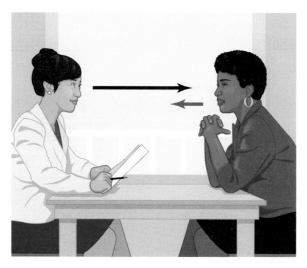

FIGURE 2-7A Clinician-centered interviewing: The clinician (pharmacist) is in control of the conversation. The patient responds to questions, indicated by the short red arrows.

Example 2

Jessica is a fourth-year pharmacy student on rotation at the outpatient care center. She is scheduled to see BJ, a 48-year-old woman with hypertension. This is the first time that Jessica is interviewing a patient. She is nervous, but she has prepared by reviewing the chart. During the chart review, she discovers that BJ's blood pressure is not at goal.

Jessica: Hello, are you BJ?

BJ: Yes.

Jessica: Ok, I have some questions about your high blood pressure, because it is not controlled.

BJ: Ok. . . .

Jessica: Do you know your goal blood pressure?

BJ: No, but I think it is supposed to be 120/80.

Jessica: How's your diet? Do you eat a lot of salt in your diet?

BJ: No. I don't put salt on my food.

Jessica: Do you take your lisinopril once a day?

BJ: Yes.

Jessica: How often do you exercise?

BJ: I exercise 3 times a week.

Jessica: Ok. That's all I need to know. I'm going to tell your doctor that I think she needs to increase your lisinopril dose, because your blood pressure is not at goal. Thank you for your time.

BJ: You're welcome.

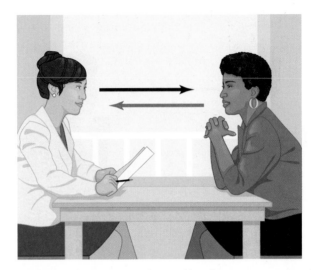

FIGURE 2-7B Patient-centered interviewing: The equal-length arrows represent a dialogue that takes place between the patient and the clinician.

Patient-centered interview:
An interview style in which the clinician creates an environment where the patient's concerns are addressed as a high priority. The patient is highly involved and engaged in the interview.

Patient-centered interviewing, on the other hand, has the patient's experience and concerns in mind (Fortin et al., 2012; Platt et al., 2001; Smith & Hoppe, 1991; Bird & Cohen-Cole, 1991). This type of interviewing method allows the patient to communicate their needs (**FIGURE 2-7B**), which are then incorporated into the care plan for the patient. Although patient-centered interviewing is a desired method to use with patients, it is still important to maintain focus. The pharmacist should make a point to address the patient's concerns while still addressing the medication-related issues that may impact patient outcomes, keeping in mind that the cause of the medication-related issues may be as a result of the patient's concerns and that resolution of the issue may occur only if the patient's concerns are incorporated into the treatment plan. Accomplishing this requires using a combination of patient-centered and clinician-centered interviewing (Smith & Hoppe, 1991; Bird & Cohen-Cole, 1991).

Fact Checking

Similar to the fact-checking step in the preparation phase, this step also involves the pharmacist asking the questions, "Does this make sense?" and "What's missing?" The pharmacist should have gathered enough information at this point to answer any of the questions that were generated during the preparation phase, identified or ruled out any drug-related problems, and addressed the purpose of the visit. In addition, the pharmacist should compare the information obtained with his or her own clinical knowledge base to determine if the patient's clinical presentation, interview responses, or concerns are congruent with what is expected or has been reported in similar situations. If there are still unanswered questions or unresolved issues, the pharmacist may gather more information or discuss the concerns with the healthcare provider.

A Culturally Competent Approach to Patient-Centered Interviewing

Using a patient-centered interviewing process will introduce information that the clinician would not have learned about using a clinician-centered interviewing approach.

Utilizing a patient-centered interviewing approach also allows for the introduction of cultural elements into the patient–pharmacist discussion. Because culture can influence healthcare-seeking practices and belief systems regarding how disease states are manifested and treated, obtaining the patient's input in regard to their medical concerns could help when creating a patient care plan.

Summary

Patient interviews are a very important part of pharmacist patient care. Effective and efficient interviews occur when the pharmacist is properly prepared. Prior to seeing the patient, the pharmacist should gather information from the patient chart, determine the pharmacist–patient relationship, and check for missing or unclear information. During the patient interview, the pharmacist can establish a relationship with the patient and gather more information that will be used in developing a drug therapy plan.

Patient-centered interviewing allows the patient to contribute more to the patient visit. Patients will be able to express their concerns, something not done during clinician-centered interviewing. Patient-centered interviewing will allow the pharmacist to gather more insight on how culture affects the patient's health beliefs, which can in turn impact how a patient prefers to be treated.

Review Questions

You are a student pharmacist at an outpatient anticoagulation clinic. Your preceptor has just received a referral for GO, a 60-year-old man who was diagnosed with deep vein thrombosis (DVT) 3 days ago. GO has been sent to the anticoagulation clinic for the management of his warfarin therapy. Your preceptor has asked you to perform a patient interview with GO while she supervises.

1. Which type of patient interview is most appropriate to conduct with GO? Why?
2. Please answer the following questions based on the dialogue in Example 2.
   a. What is your assessment of the quality of the information Jessica obtained from BJ? Please explain your answer.
   b. How could Jessica turn this encounter into a patient-centered encounter? Rewrite Jessica's portion of the script to make it more patient-centered.

References

American Society of Health-System Pharmacists. ASHP guidelines on pharmacist-conducted patient education and counseling. *Am J Health-Syst Pharm.* 1997;54:431–434.

American Society of Health-System Pharmacists. ASHP statement on the pharmacist's role in primary care. *Am J Health-Syst Pharm.* 1999;56:1665–1667.

American Society of Hospital Pharmacists. ASHP statement on pharmaceutical care. *Am J Hosp Pharm.* 1993;50:1720–1723. Available at: http://www.ashp.org/doclibrary/bestpractices /orgstpharmcare.aspx. Accessed July 18, 2013.

APhA Pharmaceutical Care Guidelines Advisory Committee 1995. *Principles of Practice for Pharmaceutical Care.* Available at: http://www.pharmacist.com/principles-practice-pharmaceutical-care. Accessed July 26, 2014.

Bird J, Cohen-Cole SA. The three-function model of the medical interview: an educational device. In: Hale M, ed. *Models of Teaching Consultation-Liaison Psychiatry*. Basel, Switzerland: Karger; 1991:65–88.

Blake K, Madhavan S, Scott V, Elswick B. Medication therapy management services in West Virginia: pharmacists' perceptions of educational and training needs. *Res Social Adm Pharm*. 2009;5(2):182–188.

Cohen-Cole SA. *The Medical Interview: The Three-Function Approach*. St. Louis, MO: Mosby-Year Book; 1991.

Fortin AH, Dwamena FC, Frankel RM, Smith RC. *Smith's Patient-Centered Interviewing: An Evidence-Based Method*. 3rd ed. New York: McGraw-Hill; 2012.

Griffith NL, Schommer JC, Wirsching RG. Survey of inpatient counseling by hospital pharmacists. *Am J Health Syst Pharm*. 1998;55:1127–1133.

Herbert K, Urmie J, Newland B, Farris K. Prediction of pharmacist intention to provide Medicare medication therapy management services using the theory of planned behavior. *Res Social Adm Pharm*. 2006;2(3):299–314.

Kaboli P, Hoth A, McClimon B, Schnipper J. Clinical pharmacists and inpatient medical care: a systematic review. *Arch Intern Med*. 2006;166(9):955–964.

Platt FW, Gaspar DL, Coulehan JL, Fox L, Adler AJ, Weston WW, et al. "Tell me about yourself": The patient-centered interview. *Ann Intern Med*. 2001;134:1079–1085.

Smith M, Bates D, Bodenheimer T, Cleary P. Why pharmacists belong in the medical home. *Health Aff*. 2010;29(5):906–913.

Smith R, Hoppe R. The patient's story: integrating the patient-and physician-centered approaches to interviewing. *Ann Intern Med*. 1991;115:470–477.

Chapter 3

Conducting a Culturally Competent Patient History

Carmita A. Coleman, PharmD, MAA

Yolanda M. Hardy, PharmD

LEARNING OBJECTIVES

At the completion of this chapter, the reader should be able to:

1. Identify the parts of the patient history.
2. Describe how each portion of the patient history applies to the pharmacist visit.
3. Describe the Kleinman, BELIEF, ETHNIC, and LEARN explanatory models.
4. Describe how incorporating explanatory models during the patient history portion of a patient interview can lead to a more culturally competent patient interaction.

KEY TERMS

Chief complaint	Medication history and allergies	Social history (SH)
Explanatory models	Past medical history (PMH)	Surgical history
Family History (FH)	Patient history	
History of present illness (HPI)	Review of systems (ROS)	

Introduction

The **patient history** is an account of the patient's experience with illnesses, disease states, medication use, or medical procedures. The purpose of the patient history is to provide an organized method for gathering the patient's information during the patient interview and relaying that information to other healthcare providers in oral or written form. Although conducting a patient history is something that all healthcare professionals perform, it is important to note that different healthcare professionals use the patient history in different ways. For example, a physician may use the patient history to help make a disease diagnosis. A pharmacist, on the other hand, may use

© antishock/Shutterstock, Inc.

Patient history:
An account of a patient's entire medical history including, but not limited to, history of medical illness, surgeries, and medication usage.

the patient history to help assess for the presence of drug-related problems and to assess drug therapy.

The patient history is the key information-gathering method used in both comprehensive and focused interviews. During a comprehensive patient interview the patient history may cover a period of years. On the other hand, the patient history conducted during a focused patient interview may span a shorter period of time, such as the time since the last visit or the time since the onset of symptoms or disease.

Elements of the Patient History

A number of areas should be covered during the patient history (**Table 3-1**). Gathering information from the patient regarding these areas will help the pharmacist have an informed view of the patient's health status, thus assisting the pharmacist in identifying

Table 3-1 Areas to Be Included in the Patient History

Areas to Cover	Why Is This Important?
Patient demographics	This information not only helps to identify the correct patient, but also provides initial information regarding the patient's current health status based on vital signs. This information may give you the first insight into drug-related problems.
Chief complaint	Often the chief complaint will indicate the main focus or purpose of the visit. It may not necessarily be a "complaint"; it may be an explanation of the reason for the referral or visit with the patient.
History of present illness	This provides more detailed information about the patient's current issue or progress since the last visit.
Past medical history	This listing of past medical illnesses may help explain the rationale for the use of certain medications or provide insight regarding the need for specialized dosing.
Family history	This information provides clues about patient risk factors for disease, thus prompting any needed screenings.
Social history	This information can help with creating a drug therapy plan that will work with the patient's lifestyle. Also, this can provide insight into current lifestyle and thus provide areas to address in terms of lifestyle modifications.
Surgical history	This listing of past surgeries may help explain the rationale for the use of certain medications or provide insight regarding the need for specialized dosing.
Medication history and allergies	This information can help with medication selection and to identify drug-related problems.
Immunization history	Pharmacists are immunizers in many locations, so knowledge of immunization history can inform the pharmacist of the need to provide vaccines.
Review of systems	Reviewing specific body systems, through either interview or physical assessment, can help provide more information about a medical condition and can help evaluate, rule out, or identify drug-related problems.

potential drug-related problems and ultimately developing a patient-specific care plan. It is important to note that a considerable amount of this information may be found in the patient's chart, and therefore can be gathered during the preparation phase of the patient interview. Information found in the chart can and should be confirmed with the patient during the interview. However, in certain situations a patient chart may not be available; in this situation, knowing the areas that should be included in the patient history will help the pharmacist gather appropriate information.

Chief Complaint

The **chief complaint** can be described as the issue that has brought the patient in to seek care from a healthcare provider. Often, the chief complaint can be ascertained by asking the patient, "What brings you in today?" A patient may answer with a response such as, "I think I have a cold," "I have terrible leg pain," or "I want to quit smoking." However, sometimes during a pharmacist–patient encounter, the chief complaint may not be so clear or it may not be a complaint at all. For example, if a patient goes to the local pharmacy to pick up medication refills and subsequently asks the pharmacist to check his blood pressure, then the patient's chief complaint isn't really a complaint; rather, it is a request for a service. As another example, a pharmacist may have been consulted by a medical team to work with a patient to help the patient improve medication adherence. In this case, her services were not sought by the patient, but rather by the healthcare provider. Therefore, another way to think about the chief complaint is as the issue that is the primary focus of the patient encounter.

Chief complaint:
A major medical or medication-related concern that results in the patient visit. Also considered the purpose of a healthcare visit.

History of Present Illness (Condition)

The **history of present illness (HPI)** is the portion of the patient history that enables the patient to elaborate more on the chief complaint. Because a patient may not have a chief complaint, the HPI can also be referred to as the history of present condition (HPC). The HPC may describe the patient's condition since the last visit or last interaction with the healthcare provider.

History of present illness (HPI):
A description of the events and symptoms related to the chief complaint.

The HPI or HPC can be formulated by asking questions related to the following areas: onset, location, duration, character, aggravating factors, relieving factors, timing, and severity. A mnemonic that can be used to remember these areas is OLD CARTS (Bickley, 2012). Another mnemonic that has been used by pharmacists to gather information during the patient interview is SCHOLAR-MAC. SCHOLAR-MAC reminds pharmacists to ask questions regarding symptoms, characteristics, history, onset, location, aggravating factors, remitting factors, medication, allergies, and other medical conditions (Leibowitz et al., 2002; Krinsky, 2012; Buring, 2007). Information obtained from each of these questioning methods is very similar. For the purposes of this text, questions asked using the OLD CARTS or SCHOLAR-MAC method will be referred to as core questions.

In addition, when the patient visit is in regard to disease state management, or if the patient's lifestyle could possibly be a contributing factor for the problem, the pharmacist should include questions regarding current lifestyle behaviors and recent lifestyle changes during the HPI or HPC.

Past Medical History

Past medical history (PMH):
A listing of a patient's past and current illnesses, which may also include information regarding onset of illness, year of diagnosis, year of disease resolution, and complications of the disease.

The **past medical history (PMH)** is the portion of the patient history that enables the pharmacist to learn about past and current medical conditions. This portion of the interview will enable the pharmacist to determine how long a person has had a current medical condition and when past medical conditions were resolved. This section can also help to identify drug-related problems. For example, when reviewing the PMH, one can anticipate which types of medications would be needed to treat the condition. The pharmacist can then check this information against what is listed in the medication list and with the patient to determine if there is a missing medication. Conversely, checking the medication list against the PMH, the pharmacist may be able to discover that the patient is taking medications for which there is no medical indication.

Family History

Family history (FH):
A listing of medical conditions that members of the patient's family have experienced. Typically includes chronic illnesses that have been experienced by 1st degree relatives or illnesses that cause an increase in hereditary risk of development.

The **family history (FH)** provides the pharmacist with information regarding medical conditions that are common in the patient's family as well as information necessary to help determine the patient's risk for disease. At the least, the FH should contain health-related information regarding the patient's mother, father, siblings, and children. Additionally, the FH should contain age and cause of death of these primary relatives, if necessary. The FH can be a valuable tool for a pharmacist for screening purposes and for providing health education to the patient.

Example

AJ, a 38-year-old African American man, has been referred to your hypertension clinic for new-onset hypertension. His PMH is significant for hypertension and seasonal allergies. This is your first time meeting AJ, so you decide to perform a comprehensive patient interview. You ask AJ about his family history during the patient history and discover that his mother and father, as well as his grandparents, have type 2 diabetes. You remember that type 2 diabetes can have a familial link, and therefore you suggest that AJ be screened for diabetes.

Social History

Social history (SH):
A description of a patient's nonmedical history. Describes information related to the patient's lifestyle and can include the patient's work history, alcohol and illicit drug use, and dietary patterns.

The **social history (SH)** is the portion of the patient history that provides the pharmacist with information regarding the patient's lifestyle. Often included in this section is the patient's use of alcohol, tobacco, and illicit drugs; however, this portion also should include information regarding the patient's diet and exercise habits, work status, and educational status. Additionally, this portion should contain information regarding the patient's living arrangements, such as if he or she lives alone or with others. This information is helpful when, for example, discussing dietary changes when the patient is not the primary provider of meals in the home, or when working with an elderly patient who may need additional caregiving assistance at home when administering medications.

Surgical History

The **surgical history** plays a limited role in the pharmacist-led patient history; however, it should not be ignored. The surgical history, as it implies, is a listing of past surgeries. Depending on the type of surgery, this information can prove valuable in helping to determine an indication for particular medications that the patient may be taking. As an example, a surgical history that includes "s/p kidney transplant" will help explain why a patient is on multiple immune-suppressing agents.

Surgical history: A listing of past surgeries. This may also include information regarding the date of the surgery and related surgical complications.

Medication History and Allergies

A pharmacist should certainly spend a considerable amount of time discussing the **medication history and allergies** portion of the patient history. Studies have shown that the medication history taken during a patient history is often incomplete. Additionally, studies have shown that patients may take herbal medications, but will not volunteer that information unless asked.

Medication history and allergies: An account of current and past medication usage. This history should include nonprescription, herbal, and home remedy usage as well as a list of medication-related allergies and the types of reactions caused by the offending agents.

When obtaining the medication history, the pharmacist should include a discussion on current and past use of prescribed medications, over-the-counter medications, vitamins, and herbal products. With each medication, vitamin, or herbal product, the pharmacist should inquire about how long the patient has taken the agent; exactly how the person is taking it, even if the person is not taking it as prescribed; and who prescribed the medication. Additionally, the pharmacist should ask the patient whether they have missed doses of the medication and whether they feel the medication is working. These two questions can be helpful in providing insight regarding the patient's adherence and their thoughts about whether they believe the medication is beneficial. Whenever possible, it is helpful to have the patient's medication bottle physically present when performing the medication history. Sharing medications with family members and loved ones often occurs; therefore, it is also important for the pharmacist to ask if the patient is taking medications that have been shared by another family member or loved one.

Knowledge of drug allergies also is an important component of the medication history. Being aware of drug allergies can help to ensure that medications the patient is allergic to are not restarted with that patient. It is important to note that patients may not understand the true meaning of a drug allergy. They may mistakenly associate an adverse effect with a drug allergy. As a result, it is important that the pharmacist follow up by asking the patient about the type of reaction they experienced when taking the offending medication.

Immunization History

Pharmacists are allowed to administer vaccines in many areas of the country. As a result, it is important for pharmacists to review the immunization history with patients. If it is discovered that the patient is due for certain vaccines, then the pharmacist can recommend or administer the vaccines to the patient. Inquiring about this information can also allow the pharmacist to provide general education to the patient about the purpose of vaccination.

Review of Systems

Review of systems (ROS):
The portion of the patient history that involves a combination of questioning and physical assessment to assess a patient's health status.

The **review of systems (ROS)** is the portion of the patient history that involves not only a series of open- and closed-ended questions, but also a physical assessment in which various measurements are taken to assess the patient's health status. In this portion of the patient history, each body system is reviewed for the presence of signs or symptoms related to the chief complaint or the primary condition for which the patient is being seen for. Healthcare providers, such as physicians or nurses, may review each body system during a patient history; however, a pharmacist typically reviews only those body systems pertinent to the purpose of the visit.

Cultural Considerations While Conducting the Patient History

It is important for pharmacists to understand not only the general impact of culture on health behaviors, but also how culture influences the individual patient's health behaviors. The patient history portion of the patient interview can be heavily influenced by a patient's culture, because culture can impact a person's way of thought, communication, value systems, relationships, rituals, traditions, and belief systems. Each of these can influence how a patient views an illness and can play a role in how the patient seeks care and chooses to treat a condition. Although the practitioner's perspective of the illness is based on the diagnosis and disease, the patient may not share this view. Therefore, a full understanding of the patient's cultural perspective regarding illness and disease gives a starting point for appropriate patient care.

It would be impossible for a pharmacist or any other healthcare professional to study and memorize the various behavior patterns, beliefs, and values of every culture. Rather, a more realistic way of learning about the cultural influence on health behaviors is by using various methods that will enable the patient to talk about beliefs during the process of performing the patient history. **Explanatory models** have been designed to include behaviors and information-gathering techniques that allow for open communication between the healthcare provider and patient. Use of explanatory models during the patient interview helps to elicit the patient's experience and beliefs regarding the illness and treatment of the illness. These models can help the healthcare professional have more of a patient-centered interview and obtain more information about the patient's perspective, including experiences, beliefs, values, and feelings, regarding their illness. These models easily integrate into the patient interview format previously discussed and should be with every patient, regardless of cultural background. Pharmacists will find the explanatory models very useful when performing the HPI or HPC, as well as the medication history.

Explanatory models:
A method used when describing a rationale for how or why events happen. Can be utilized during patient interviews to gather an understanding of the patient's beliefs on how or why an illness developed and how and why an illness should be treated.

A number of models have been created to assist clinicians in gathering information in a manner that enables one to learn about the patient's cultural beliefs and practices, and thus incorporate them into the care plan for the patient. Two models, the LEARN (**Table 3-2**) and RESPECT (**Table 3-3**) models, provide a framework for communication between clinicians and patients based on behaviors that should be demonstrated by the healthcare provider during the patient visit.

Table 3-2 LEARN Model

L–Listen	The clinician should elicit the patient's perspective of the illness, including feelings about the illness and preferences regarding treatment, in an empathetic manner.
E–Explain	The clinician should communicate to the patient his or her own explanation of the illness and treatment based on clinical knowledge. The clinician should be open in the explanation, even when the actual cause or diagnosis may not be known. This explanation should be provided in a manner that can be understood by the patient.
A–Acknowledge	The patient and clinician together acknowledge the similarities and differences of their perspectives related to the illness and treatment. The clinician and patient should attempt to find a common agreement with the differences.
R–Recommend	The clinician recommendations and plan for management of the illness include patient involvement and address patient concerns.
N–Negotiate	Together, the patient and clinician develop a treatment plan that is acceptable to all. The key is that the plan has mutual agreement.

Data from Berlin EA, Fowkes Jr, WC. A teaching framework for cross-cultural health care. *West J Med.* 1983;139:934–938.

Table 3-3 RESPECT Model

R–Respect	Connect on a social level. Seek the patient's point of view. Consciously attempt to suspend judgment. Recognize and avoid making assumptions.
E–Empathy	Remember that the patient has come to you for help. Seek out and understand the patient's rationale for his or her behaviors or illness. Verbally acknowledge and legitimize the patient's feelings.
S–Support	Ask about and try to understand barriers to care and compliance. Help the patient overcome barriers. Involve family members, if appropriate. Reassure the patient you are and will be available to help.
P–Partnership	Be flexible with regard to issues of control. Negotiate roles when necessary. Stress that you will be working together to address medical problems.
E–Explanations	Check often for understanding. Use verbal clarification techniques.
C–Cultural competence	Respect the patient and his or her culture and beliefs. Understand that the patient's view of you may be identified by ethnic or cultural stereotypes. Be aware of your own biases or preconceptions. Know your limitations in addressing medical issues across cultures. Know your personal style and recognize when it may not be working with a given patient.
T–Trust	Self-disclosure may be an issue for some patients who are not accustomed to Western medical approaches. Take the necessary time and consciously work to establish trust.

Data from Welch M. *Enhancing Awareness and Improving Cultural Competence in Health Care. A Partnership Guide for Teaching Diversity and Cross-Cultural Concepts in Health Professional Training.* San Francisco: University of California at San Francisco; 1998.

The LEARN model, developed by Drs. Berlin and Fowkes (1983), describes a communication approach that enables the patient to express his or her perspective on the disease and its management, thus allowing the clinician to understand the patient's perspective. Initially this model was used by medical residents to understand multicultural populations and overcome barriers of difference; however, it can be of value during pharmacist-led patient interviews. The pharmacist could utilize this model not only when learning more about the patient's perspective on disease, but also to help learn more about the patient's perspective on medication use for treatment of disease. The LEARN model is intended to supplement the patient history portion of the interview by adding an explanation to the patient's rationale of illness; however, information gained from the patient's explanation should then be incorporated into the treatment plan.

The RESPECT model, developed by Welch (1998), focuses on the development of a therapeutic relationship with the patient. To adequately apply this method, enough time must be spent developing a rapport with the patient. Therefore, this could be a model used when seeing patients for multiple follow-up visits. It also stresses the importance of meeting patients' desires and lending support. Finally, an element of introspection also is necessary with this model. To effectively use this model, the healthcare provider should identify his or her own underlying attitudes and biases toward beliefs regarding culturally influenced healthcare practices.

Three additional models, BELIEF, ETHNIC, and Kleinman's Eight Questions, provide useful examples of questions to ask during a patient interview and can augment the core questions used to gather information. With each model, a question or statement is asked of the patient to determine their perspective of the various factors. Pharmacists can use each of the models as designed or can modify the questions when discussing medication therapy with patients.

The BELIEF model (**Table 3-4**) was created by Dobbie and colleagues (2003) as a cultural interviewing tool for use by medical students with limited clinical knowledge; however, this model can be beneficial for other healthcare professional students and trained practitioners as well. This model helps to gather information on the patient's beliefs not only in regard to the origins of the illness, but also about the illness as well as the patient's ideas on how the illness is affecting life. It is important to differentiate this model, which describes an interviewing technique, from the health belief model, which is used to predict health behaviors.

The ETHNIC model (**Table 3-5**) was created by Levin and colleagues (2000) and is applicable to a variety of cultures in determining beliefs. In addition to gathering information about the patient's beliefs, this model also allows the clinician to learn about the patient's views on various treatment-seeking practices and beliefs. The ETHNIC model also allows for the patient to play a role in treatment-making decisions.

Understanding the impact of culture on health seeking and adherence practices early on, Kleinman and colleagues (Kleinman, 1980; Kleinman, Eisenburg, & Good, 1978) developed the Eight Questions model in the late 1970s (**Table 3-6**). These questions were designed to elicit the patient's feelings and beliefs about sickness, in addition to ascertaining

Table 3-4 BELIEF Model

	BELIEF Questions	Modified for Pharmacists
B–Health beliefs	What do you think is the cause of your illness? Do you have any folk or over-the-counter (OTC) remedies for your condition? Do you or your family have any spiritual beliefs about your illness?	What do you think is the cause of your illness? Do you have any folk or OTC remedies for your condition? Do you or your family have any spiritual beliefs about your illness? *Do you believe that medication is the best way to treat this condition?*
E–Explanation	Why do you think it happened at this time? How do you explain your illness? Do you believe that you did anything to cause your illness?	Why do you think it happened at this time? How do you explain your illness? Do you believe that you did anything to cause your illness? *Why do you think the medication (or dose) changed this time? Do you believe that you need the medication? Why or why not? Do you believe that you did anything to cause the medication change?*
L–Learn	Describe your belief or opinion of your illness. What can I do to best help you?	Describe your belief or opinion of your illness. What can I do to best help you? *Describe your belief or opinion of using this medication.*
I–Impact	How is this illness impacting your life? What is your most prominent problem that you are experiencing as a result of your illness? How is your family handling this problem?	How is this illness impacting your life? What is your most prominent problem that you are experiencing as a result of your illness? How is your family handling this problem? *How does using this medication(s) impact your life? What is the most prominent problem that you are experiencing as a result of using this medication?*
E–Empathy	I understand that this must be very difficult for you. Is there something I can do to make this easier for you? Many people feel as you do.	I understand that this must be very difficult for you. Is there something I can do to make this easier for you? Many people feel as you do.
F–Feelings	Describe how you feel about your illness. What do you fear most about your illness? What is troubling you at this time?	Describe how you feel about your illness. What do you fear most about your illness? What is troubling you at this time? *Describe how you feel about using medication. What do you fear most about using medication? What is troubling you about using this medication?*

*Italicized questions have been modified for pharmacists

Data from Dobbie AE, Medrano M, Tysinger J, Olney C. The BELIEF instrument: A preclinical teaching tool to elicit patients' health beliefs. *Fam Med.* 2003;35:316–319.

Table 3-5 ETHNIC Model

	ETHNIC Model Questions	Modified for Pharmacists
E–Explanation	How do you explain your illness? Have you heard or seen any information about your illness?	How do you explain your illness? Have you heard or seen any information about your illness?
T–Treatment	What treatments have you tried for your illness? Is there anything that you do or do not eat or drink to stay healthy?	What treatments have you tried for your illness? Is there anything that you do or do not eat or drink to stay healthy? *Have you tried any medications, vitamins, or herbal products? Are there home remedies to treat this?*
H–Healers	Who else has helped you with your illness? Have you gotten advice from alternative or folk medicine for your illness?	Who else has helped you with your illness? Have you gotten advice from alternative or folk medicine for your illness?
N–Negotiate	What can I do to help you the most? What do you feel are the best options for you?	What can I do to help you the most? What do you feel are the best options for you? *Do you think this is best treated with medication? With this medication? Why or why not?*
I–Intervention	Based on the options that you have suggested, let's agree on a few.	Based on the options that you have suggested, let's agree on a few.
C–Collaborate	How can we work together on this? Who else needs to be included on our treatment plan?	How can we work together on this? Who else needs to be included on our treatment plan?

*Italicized questions have been modified for pharmacists

Data from Levin SJ, Like RC, Gottlieb JE. ETHNIC: A framework for culturally competent clinical practice. In: Appendix: Useful clinical interviewing mnemonics. *Patient Care.* 2000;34:188–189.

how the patient believes the disease will progress and what the patient's expectations are from treatment. This model also helps the clinician learn more about the patient's experience with the condition, as well as fears related to the condition.

Each of the aforementioned models can be used when working with any patient. Depending on the practice setting and pharmacist–patient relationship, one model may prove to be more useful than another. In certain instances a combination of multiple models may need to be used to gather the information needed from the patient. Patients are very perceptive and can easily determine when the practitioner is using a script to elicit a response. Therefore, practitioners should become comfortable when using a particular model or models, individualizing it to their practice and the situation.

Table 3-6 Kleinman Explanatory Model

Kleinman Questions	Modified for Pharmacists
1. What do you call the problem?	1. What do you call the problem?
2. What do you think has caused the problem?	2. What do you think has caused the problem?
3. Why do you think it started when it did?	3. Why do you think it started when it did?
4. What do you think the sickness does? How does it work?	4. What do you think the sickness does? How does it work? *What do you think this medication does? How does it work?*
5. How severe is the sickness? Will it have a long or short course?	5. How severe is the sickness? Will it have a long or short course? *How long do you think you would have to take the medication for this?*
6. What kind of treatment do you think you should receive?	6. What kind of treatment do you think you should receive? *Do you think this is best treated with medication? With this medication? Why or why not?*
7. What are the chief problems the sickness has caused?	7. What are the chief problems the sickness has caused? *What problems do you think this medication will cause?*
8. What do you fear most about the sickness?	8. What do you fear most about the sickness? *What do you fear most about this medication?*

*Italicized questions have been modified for pharmacists

Data from Kleinman A. *Patients and Healers in the Context of Culture.* Berkeley: University of California Press; 1980.

In addition to aiding in the information-gathering process, explanatory models are also of use when developing a treatment plan. Explanatory models allow for negotiation and eventual integration of the patient's understanding and desires regarding the diagnosis and treatment into the plan, thus allowing the patient to take more of a role in the decision-making process regarding how to treat the illness (Kleinman, 1978, 1980).

Summary

The patient history is the portion of the patient interview that allows the pharmacist to gather information from the patient. This information will provide the pharmacist with insight into the patient's experience with a disease or condition. Culture is integral to health care and, consequently, to the healthcare encounter. The use of patient-centered, culturally appropriate care models is essential to a successful patient assessment. Eliciting the patient's perceptions and beliefs can shape the relationship between practitioner and patient. Overall, each model stresses the acknowledgment of and respect for the patient's voice regarding the choice of healthcare services. The use of the model moves the relationship beyond the biomedical and into the realm of psychosocial constructs. It demands that the practitioner exhibit care as part of the clinical encounter. In addition, it demands that the patient be an active participant. Regardless of the explanatory model of communication used, practitioner comfort leads to a better interaction. Patients are required to express their needs, and the practitioner is required to incorporate those preferences into the care plan. True negotiation necessitates that the practitioner relinquish control of the healthcare encounter. Researchers have developed models that range from a simple overlay during the history taking to a more involved, repeated inquiry about patient preferences and needs. In the end, knowing the patient more intimately and negotiating a final plan is done in an effort to improve patient outcomes.

Review Questions

1. A patient has been referred to you for medication nonadherence. The primary care provider does not understand why the patient refuses to take his medication as prescribed. Explain how use of the explanatory model will help in understanding the patient's rationale for not taking the medication.
2. You are the pharmacist on duty at the local community pharmacy. DC, a 50-year-old man, comes to you complaining of a cough and is seeking treatment. Create a list of questions that you would ask DC in order to get an accurate history of his present condition (HPC).

References

Berlin EA, Fowkes Jr, WC. A teaching framework for cross-cultural health care. *West J Med.* 1983;139:934–938.

Bickley LS, Szilagyi PG, Bates B. *Bates' Guide to Physical Examination and History Taking.* 11th ed. Philadelphia, PA: Wolters Kluwer Health/Lippincott Williams & Wilkins; 2012.

Buring S, Kirby J, Conrad W. A structured approach for teaching students to counsel self-care patients. *Am J Pharm Educ.* 2007;71(1):8.

Dobbie AE, Medrano M, Tysinger J, Olney C. The BELIEF instrument: a preclinical teaching tool to elicit patients' health beliefs. *Fam Med.* 2003;35:316–319.

Kleinman A. *Patients and Healers in the Context of Culture.* Berkeley: University of California Press; 1980.

Kleinman AM, Eisenburg L, Good B. Culture, illness, and care: clinical lessons from anthropologic and cross-cultural research. *Ann Intern Med.* 1978;88:251–258.

Krinsky D, Berardi R, Ferreri S, Hume A, Newton G, Rollins C, et al. *Handbook of Nonprescription Drugs: An Interactive Approach to Self-Care.* 17th ed. Washington, DC: American Pharmacists Association; 2012.

Leibowitz K, Ginsburg D. Counseling self-treating patients quickly and effectively. Proceedings of the APhA Inaugural Self-Care Institute; May 17–19, 2002.

Levin SJ, Like RC, Gottlieb JE. ETHNIC: A framework for culturally competent clinical practice. In: Appendix: Useful clinical interviewing mnemonics. *Patient Care.* 2000;34:188–189.

Warren NS. Cultural and spiritual mnemonic tools for use in genetic counseling. Available at: http://www.geneticcounselingtoolkit.com/pdf_files/Cultural%20and%20Spiritual%20 Mnemonic%20Tools%2011.06.09.pdf. Accessed March 31, 2013.

Welch M. *Enhancing Awareness and Improving Cultural Competence in Health Care. A Partnership Guide for Teaching Diversity and Cross-Cultural Concepts in Health Professional Training.* San Francisco: University of California at San Francisco; 1998.

Unit III

The Culturally Competent Physical Assessment

The idea of a pharmacist performing a physical assessment may bring a sense of hesitation to some practitioners, because it may seem like the pharmacist is crossing practice boundaries into an area historically reserved for nurses and physicians. However, with the added responsibilities of pharmacists in the practice of patient care, understanding the role of the physical assessment and having the ability to perform a physical assessment are imperative.

There are three main reasons why a pharmacist should have the ability to perform a physical assessment (FIGURE UIII-1). Performance of various physical assessment skills can help the pharmacist triage in the outpatient setting. Findings from assessing the patient, which include both the patient interview and performance of physical assessment skills, can help the pharmacist discern if a patient's symptoms can be treated with over-the-counter agents should be addressed with the patient's primary care provider, or warrant immediate emergency treatment.

Performing a physical assessment can help the pharmacist discover or assess adverse drug events. As drug experts, pharmacists are aware of the adverse drug

---

Reasons for Pharmacists to Perform Physical Assessments
1) Help to determine if a patient's condition can be managed by self-care treatment or warrants care from a healthcare professional.
2) Can assist in discovering or assessing adverse drug events.
3) Can assist in assessing therapeutic outcomes of drug therapy.

FIGURE UIII-1 Reasons for pharmacists to perform physical assessments.

© onidslock/Shutterstock, Inc.

events of many prescription and nonprescription medications. Due to various reasons, a patient or other healthcare professional may not notice that a clinical condition is the result of an adverse drug reaction. Pharmacists can be proactive and assess patients for the development of various signs and symptoms related to an adverse drug event.

A major responsibility of the pharmacist in providing patient care is to ensure positive therapeutic outcomes for the patient. Performing skills such as measuring a patient's blood pressure can help determine if a recent dose increase of a hypertensive medication is effective.

Unit III of this text discusses physical assessment skills that are pertinent to the practice of pharmacy. The chapters in this unit first discuss the clinical presentation of various disease processes, followed by a discussion of questions to ask during the patient interview, instructions for performing the physical assessment when this is necessary, and a discussion of the findings. Each chapter will also include a discussion of the clinical presentation of drug-induced processes and assessment skills that can be performed in discovering or assessing the drug-induced condition. Finally, each chapter will close with a discussion of cultural elements that should be taken into consideration with the assessment.

Chapter 4

Mental Status and Behavior Assessment

Mark D. Watanabe, PharmD, PhD, BCPP

LEARNING OBJECTIVES

At the completion of this chapter, the reader should be able to:

1. List important assessment tools used to determine the mental status of an individual during a clinical interview.

2. Determine appropriate questions to ask individuals when performing a mental status examination.

3. Explain the role of self-assessment questionnaires in the screening process for psychiatric disorders.

4. List drugs that may cause adverse side effects that mimic psychiatric symptoms.

5. Determine appropriate questions to ask individuals when performing a Cultural Formulation Interview in psychiatry.

KEY TERMS

Affect

Appearance

Behavior

Cognitive function

Cultural Formulation Interview (CFI)

Mental status examination (MSE)

Mood

Patient Health Questionnaire (PHQ)

Perceptions

Speech

Thought content

Thought process

Introduction

Assessments of mental status and behavior are essential to the diagnosis of psychiatric disorders as well as other medical conditions that may involve changes in mental status or behavior. The standard clinical interview is expanded to include additional questions specifically intended to probe for the presence of symptoms accompanied by significant distress and poor functioning that may warrant overt treatment. Unlike other tools that

© MikeF/Shutterstock, Inc.

Mental status examination (MSE): Foundational semi-structured interview used to identify patient-specific target symptoms addressed in an individualized treatment plan.

rely extensively on more objective measures, the semi-structured approaches described in this chapter require the user to have a high capacity for listening and observation. Pharmacists who possess this particular skill set could be well-poised to serve as triage agents for appropriate referral.

This chapter will first review some of the core assessments utilized in identifying key symptomatology that would appear in a psychiatric treatment plan independent of cultural perspectives. Some examples of where cultural awareness and sensitivity may impact the actual diagnosis will be provided. Finally, an overview of the American Psychiatric Association's cultural formulation process, as suggested in the current edition of the *Diagnostic and Statistical Manual of Mental Disorders*, 5th ed. (DSM-5), will follow.

Appearance: Assessed by the mental status examination; an individual's dress, grooming, and personal hygiene.

Clinical Presentation: Mental Status Changes

Any observed alteration in mental status or behavior that constitutes a variation from a usual or baseline pattern would likely prompt an assessment. An initial physical evaluation should always be performed first in order to rule out any medical causes for the change. Some somatic symptoms that are medically unexplained may be attributed to a psychiatric etiology instead. In fact, physical or somatic complaints are commonly reported in patients with depression and anxiety, two of the more common psychiatric diagnoses a pharmacist might encounter in community or ambulatory care practice. Disturbances in sleep patterns, fatigue or psychomotor agitation, and fluctuations in weight or appetite are part of the usual constellation of symptoms seen in both depressive and anxiety disorders. The presence of these clinical events, when associated with concurrent and significant impairment in daily functioning, would inform a recommendation of a referral for a more thorough behavioral health evaluation.

Behavior: Assessed by the mental status examination; particular attention is paid to posture and body movements.

The Patient Interview

Speech: Assessed by the mental status examination; focus is placed on describing the quantity, rate, and volume of speech as well as the fluency of language and the ability to articulate words.

The patient interview, known as the **mental status examination (MSE)** is the foundation of the assessment process and is used to identify patient-specific target symptoms that may need to be addressed in the overall treatment plan (American Psychiatric Association, 2006). It consists of five general domains to be evaluated:

- **Appearance** and **behavior**
- **Speech** and language
- **Mood** and **affect**
- Thoughts and **perceptions**
- **Cognitive function:** attention, memory, information and vocabulary, abstract thinking, calculations, and constructional ability

Mood: Assessed by the mental status examination; pervasive and sustained emotion.

The execution of the MSE relies on the standard combination of asking questions and making observations, and may even be initiated by simple inquiries such as "How are you doing today?" Examples of the discrete areas to be covered by the clinical examiner that may be included are provided in **Table 4-1**.

Table 4-1 Components of the Mental Status Examination

Domain	Observations	Questions to Consider
Appearance and behavior	Assess the patient's level of consciousness[1]	Is the patient awake and alert? Does the patient understand your questions? Does the patient respond appropriately and reasonably?
	Assess the patient's posture and motor behavior[1]	How would you characterize the patient's posture and motor behavior? How would you describe the pace, range, and character of body movements (e.g., calm, nervous)?
	Assess the patient's dress, grooming, and personal hygiene[1]	How is the patient dressed? How well are hair, nails, teeth, and skin groomed? How do these areas compare with those of other people of comparable age, lifestyle, and socioeconomic group?
	Assess the patient's facial expressions[1]	Are expressions appropriate? Is the face relatively immobile throughout the interview? Is it overly animated?
	Assess the patient's manner, affect, and relationship to people and things[1]	Does the affect reflect the mood or does it seem inappropriate or extreme at times? Does the affect vary appropriately with topics under discussion? How would you describe the patient regarding openness, approachability, and reactions to others?
Speech and language	Assess the quantity of speech[1]	Does the patient tend to be verbal or silent? Are the patient's comments spontaneous or only offered in response to direct questions?
	Assess the rate of speech[1]	Is the speech fast or slow?
	Assess the volume of speech[1]	Is the speech soft or loud?
	Assess the articulation of words[1]	Does the patient speak distinctly and clearly?
	Assess the fluency of language[1]	Is the rate and flow of speaking smooth, or are there hesitancies and gaps? Does the content make sense?

Affect: Assessed by the mental status examination; how a person expresses a subjectively experienced emotion.

Perceptions: Assessed by the mental status examination; characterization of how an individual experiences real external stimuli.

Cognitive function: Assessed by the mental status examination; domains assessed include orientation, attention, memory, learning ability, and problem solving.

(continues)

Table 4-1 Components of the Mental Status Examination (*continued*)

Domain	Observations	Questions to Consider
Mood and affect	Assess the patient's own perception of her or his mood[2]	How good or bad has the patient felt emotionally (i.e., mood)? How long has the patient's mood been this way? How intense has the feeling been? Has the mood been stable or labile? Is the mood appropriate to the patient's circumstances? Is how the patient expresses her or his mood (affect) appropriate?
Thoughts and perceptions	Assess the patient's **thought processes** as reflected in her or his words and speech[1]	Does the content of speech progress logically toward a goal or is it scattered? Is the conversation logical, organized, relevant, and coherent?
	Assess the patient's **thought content**[1]	Does the patient experience and express particular fears, obsessions, compulsions, feelings of unreality or depersonalization, or delusions (fixed false beliefs)?
	Assess the patient's perceptions[2]	How does the patient experience real external stimuli (perceptions)? Does the patient experience any subjective sensory perceptions that are not based in reality (e.g., hallucinations)?
	Assess the patient's insight and judgment[2]	Does the patient acknowledge and understand the reasons for the current clinic or hospital visit? Can the patient offer reasonable and mature responses to various situations (e.g., regarding family or social interactions, employment, finances, or interpersonal conflicts)?
Cognitive function	Assess the patient's orientation[2]	Is the patient oriented to person, place, and time?
	Assess the patient's attention[2]	Can the patient repeat a string of numbers after one is provided? Is the patient able to serially subtract 7s, starting from 100? Can the patient spell simple words backward?

Thought process: Assessed by the mental status examination; description of the logical flow, organization, or coherence of ideas and thoughts as expressed by an individual.

Thought content: Assessed by the mental status examination; determination of the presence of unusual thinking or feelings of detachment from reality.

Table 4-1 Components of the Mental Status Examination (*continued*)

Domain	Observations	Questions to Consider
	Assess the patient's remote memory[2]	Is the patient able to recall birthdays, anniversaries, jobs held, or events relevant to the patient's past?
	Assess the patient's recent memory[2]	Is the patient able to recall any current events or recent activities accurately?
	Assess the patient's new learning ability[2]	Is the patient able to remember new information introduced earlier in the interview?
	Assess the patient's higher cognitive functioning[2]	Is the patient able to respond accurately to tests of information and vocabulary, calculating ability, abstract thinking, and constructional ability?

[1]Assessed by active listening or direct observation
[2]Assessed by directly asking questions or requesting tasks of patient

Data from Snyderman D, Rovner BW. Mental status exam in primary care: a review. *Am Fam Physician*. 2009;80(8):809–814.

The results obtained from the MSE can serve multiple purposes, depending on the clinical setting. In psychiatry, it is the primary instrument used to identify the symptoms that inform both formal diagnosis and treatment plans for a particular patient. The MSE is used less frequently in the primary care setting, but elements of it may be incorporated into the standard clinical interview in order to assess the need to refer the patient to specialty behavioral health care. An interview resulting in the discovery of disorders of mood or thought process will be more likely to require such a referral. The clinician should try to determine the presence of any negative stigma a given individual may associate with mental illness in order to frame questions in a sensitive and respectful manner. **Table 4-2** reviews the importance of specific elements of the mental status examination in clinical practice.

In cases where the patient and the treating clinician do not share the same cultural and socioeconomic background, additional efforts should be made to acknowledge those differences so that an appropriate evaluation may take place. Otherwise, misunderstandings and inaccurate perceptions on the part of the clinician may result in greater potential for misdiagnosis. For instance, if a patient reports a belief in witchcraft or having conversations with God, it may not necessarily reflect the presence of delusions or auditory hallucinations; rather, it may be a normative construct in the culture of origin. In other cases, it may be appropriate to expand the MSE to include inquiries into the physical well-being of the individual because some cultures may explain psychiatric symptoms with a greater emphasis on somatic complaints (e.g., headaches, stomach upset, sleep disturbances, nervousness, inability to concentrate, trembling). There may even be culture-specific terms

Table 4-2 Information Gathered from the Mental Status Examination

Level of consciousness	Assess for capacity to respond and the reliability of responses
Posture and motor behavior	Assess for symptoms (e.g., catatonia) or abnormal movements (e.g., medication-induced extrapyramidal symptoms)
Grooming and hygiene	Assess capacity to maintain activities of daily living
Facial expressions	Assess current status of affect and mood, and whether they are congruent
Quantity, rate, and volume of speech	Assess for presence of potential medication-responsive target symptoms (e.g., pressured speech)
Fluency of language	Assess for either cognitive impairment or thought disorder consistent with a particular psychiatric diagnosis (e.g., schizophrenia)
Perception of mood	Assist in the identification and characterization of specific mood symptoms (e.g., depression or mania) as targets of treatment
Thought processes	Assess for the presence of thought disorders symptomatic of a psychiatric disorder
Thought content	Assess for the presence of unusual thought content reflective of a specific psychiatric disorder (e.g., schizophrenia, depression, bipolar disorder)
Sensory perceptions	Assess for the presence of hallucinations (i.e., perceptions not based in reality)
Insight and judgment	Assist in determining likelihood of adherence to recommended treatment regimen
Cognitive function	Evaluate for cognitive impairment that could be secondary to a psychiatric/medical disorder or an undesired effect of medication

for distress that may be shared during the interview (e.g., "attack of nerves," "thinking too much," "sent sickness," "evil eye," "soul loss") that may indicate underlying disorders requiring treatment.

Psychiatric Self-Assessment Tools

There are self-administered assessments that a clinician might facilitate for a patient in general ambulatory care practice. The goal of these scales, presented in patient-appropriate language, is to determine whether a patient exhibits an array of symptoms meeting a threshold severity sufficient to warrant a more thorough psychiatric evaluation. As such, these are screening, not diagnostic, tools.

The Patient Health Questionnaire (PHQ)

For approximately two decades, one resource used by primary care providers in the screening for psychiatric disorders has been the PRIME-MD (Primary Care Evaluation of

Case #1

AA is a 25-year-old woman who presents to the behavioral health clinic after being recently discharged from the state hospital with a diagnosis of schizophrenia. You are assigned to take a medication history from her. She is well-groomed and her appearance is consistent with her chronological age. Her voice is soft but audible. Eye contact with you is good and her speech is understandable. There are no reports of depression or anxiety. She denies hearing voices and states that she has been taking her medication regularly after leaving the hospital. You would like to assess her cognitive skills to check for both resolution of her symptoms and potential emergence of adverse medication-related side effects.

Questions

1. What clinical tool can be used to evaluate this?
2. What are some examples of specific questions that could be asked of AA?

Mental Disorders) checklist and the **Patient Health Questionnaire (PHQ)** that was subsequently derived from it. These procedures were developed by Spitzer et al. (1994; with an educational grant by Pfizer, Inc.) and can assist the clinician in recognizing common mental health problems encountered in primary care (i.e., anxiety, depression, alcohol dependence, eating disorders, and psychosomatic symptoms). The original PRIME-MD consisted of a one-page, 26-item questionnaire in which a patient would simply indicate the presence or absence of symptoms associated with each of the problem categories in the past month. The full PHQ consolidates some of these items and asks the patient to more fully characterize any current problems regarding their severity and how long each has persisted.

The nine items assessed in Question 2 can also be administered separately as the PHQ-9, which specifically screens for depression. In this case, numerical scores are attached to the associated severity ratings (on a 0–3 scale); total scores greater than 10 would most likely indicate a need to initiate a specific treatment plan for treating depression with

Patient Health Questionnaire (PHQ): Self-rating scale used by patients as a screening tool for emerging symptoms of depression.

Case #2

BL is a 52-year-old man who visited his primary care provider for several months with complaints of aches and pains in his joints and back. His symptoms had not improved despite numerous trials of commonly used analgesics, so he was referred to a behavioral health clinic for a psychiatric evaluation to rule out depression. After missing three initial scheduled appointments, BL finally appeared and was visibly upset about having to be seen at a "crazy clinic" for pain. The intake interview revealed that BL had recently immigrated with his family to the United States only a year ago and he has had difficulty finding work because of his limited ability to speak English. When asked what was the most important concern for him at the present time, he answered: "To find job to help family and find safe new home where shootings do not happen."

Question

1. What cultural issues may need to be considered as BL is being assessed for a potential diagnosis of depression?

psychotherapy and/or pharmacotherapy. Other self-rating scales for depression screening include the Beck Depression Inventory (Beck & Steer, 1984) and the Zung Self-Rating Scale (Zung, 1965). For more visually oriented individuals, a Likert scale similar to those used in pain assessment may be used to determine the state of someone's mood. Such a scale would illustrate a smiling face at one end of a line and a face with a sad, tearful expression at the other end, and the person is to indicate with an "X" where on the linear continuum their current feelings lie.

It is important to always probe for the risk of potential suicide in every patient who undergoes a mental status evaluation. Because many tools have not incorporated cultural variations into these suicide risk assessments, Chu et al. (2010, 2013) have developed a cultural model of suicide (which includes cultural sanctions, idioms of distress, minority stress, and social discord factors) and an associated Cultural Assessment of Risk for Suicide (CARS) measure to use with the usual normative procedures. If any expression of suicidal ideation or plan emerges, this invokes the highest level of concern and an immediate referral should be made.

The CAGE Test

Some behaviors exhibited by individuals may suggest the presence of an addiction related to a substance use disorder. A commonly used tool to assess this possibility is the CAGE test, where CAGE is an acronym that relates to elements of the four following questions:

1. Have you ever felt you should **C**ut down your use of drugs or alcohol?
2. Have you ever been **A**nnoyed when people have commented on your use?
3. Have you ever felt **G**uilty or badly about your use?
4. Have you ever used drugs or alcohol to **E**ase withdrawal symptoms, or to avoid feeling low after using?

Each "yes" answer scores as one point; the risk ranges from a total score of 0 to 4. It is used as a screening tool only; the results alone do not constitute sufficient evidence for making the formal diagnosis of a substance addiction disorder. An affirmative response to any of the questions may prompt many clinicians to make a referral to an addictions specialist for further evaluation.

Clinical Presentation of Drug-Induced Processes

Whenever unusual mental status changes develop in an individual, any potential primary causes such as concurrent medical conditions or unintended side effects from medication should be ruled out before making a formal diagnosis of an idiopathic psychiatric disorder. Pharmacists can provide valuable insight into this assessment by obtaining and reviewing a complete medication history. Table 4-3 lists examples of medications that have been reported to induce depressive symptoms that are indistinguishable from those found in people who are diagnosed with idiopathic major depressive disorder.

In addition, many street drugs (e.g., amphetamines, cocaine, phencyclidine [PCP], lysergic acid diethylamide [LSD]) used by individuals with documented substance abuse and dependence histories may cause psychotic symptoms such as hallucinations or delusions, which may mimic or exacerbate the clinical presentation found in schizophrenia spectrum disorders. Clinicians should be aware that a high rate of comorbidities exists

Table 4-3 Examples of Medications That May Induce Depression

Cardiovascular drugs	Beta blockers
	Clonidine
	Methyldopa
	Reserpine
Central nervous system drugs	Barbiturates
	Ethanol
	Varenicline
Other drugs	Anabolic steroids
	Corticosteroids
	Efavirenz
	Interferon
	Isotretinoin
	Levetiracetam
	Progestin
	Tamoxifen

Data from DiPiro JT, Talbert RL, Yee GC, Matzke GR, Wells BG, Posey LM, eds. *Pharmacotherapy: a Pathophysiologic Approach*. 8th ed. New York: McGraw-Hill; 2011.

between substance use disorders and other diagnoses of major mental illnesses in DSM-5. Many individuals may actually be using street drugs to "self-medicate" themselves to alleviate untreated symptoms due to an underlying psychiatric illness.

Cultural Considerations

The assessment of psychiatric disorders, which occur worldwide across cultures, requires a particular sensitivity to a number of contextual issues. Because of the increasing cultural diversity in highly developed nations, the importance of understanding the influences outside of normative Western biomedical constructs that may impact effective mental health treatment cannot be minimized. In 2001, the U.S. Office of the Surgeon General issued a supplemental report, *Mental Health: Culture, Race, and Ethnicity*, that acknowledged the significant disparities in mental health care offered to individuals of racial and ethnic minorities compared with whites. To the extent that such disparities, including access to and availability of appropriate services, may be due to limited cultural competency on the part of clinicians, there is a growing need for developing more comprehensive assessment tools that meet the needs of these underserved populations.

The establishment of a trusting therapeutic relationship between a clinician and a patient is the critical foundation for any assessment of mental health and behavior. If there is a cultural difference within this dyad, it may be helpful to enlist the assistance of a well-trained intermediary (i.e., an interpreter who is highly familiar with the native language and/or culture of the patient). If an interpreter is used to overcome barriers due to differing languages, it is also essential that the words of the patient be translated verbatim as much as possible. Because unusual verbal comments may themselves indicate the presence of a psychiatric disorder, avoidance of a filtered interpretation that "makes more sense" will help to bring those symptoms of interest to light.

The American Psychiatric Association's DSM-5 is a standard reference that defines the specific criteria for diagnosing psychiatric disorders through careful patient assessments. This most recent edition, released in 2013, emphasizes the importance of understanding the cultural context of the mental illness experience for effective clinical management. The DSM-5 recommends a systematic review of the following domains as part of a formal outline for cultural formulation:

- Cultural identity of the individual
- Cultural conceptualization of distress
- Psychosocial stressors and cultural features of vulnerability and resilience
- Cultural features of the relationship between the individual and the clinician
- Overall cultural assessment

Cultural Formulation Interview (CFI): Instrument introduced in the DSM-5 to account for potential cultural differences in definitions of the mental health problem, perceptions of causes, differences in values regarding coping mechanisms, and help seeking.

To discern the impact of cultural context on the appropriate assessment of an individual's clinical presentation as well as the clinical treatment plan, the DSM-5 offers the Cultural Formulation Interview (CFI), a 16-item instrument formulated as a semi-structured interview that may be incorporated into a standard clinical evaluation. It may be particularly useful whenever there are challenges in diagnostic assessment due to differences in the cultural, religious, or socioeconomic backgrounds of the clinician and the individual being assessed—especially when there is ambiguity regarding the match of culturally distinctive symptoms with established diagnostic criteria. An overview of the CFI is provided in **Table 4-4**.

The assessment and subsequent management of psychiatric symptoms and behavior should be implemented with great care and sensitivity to the profound stigma that is often associated with mental illness across cultures. Because of this stigma, psychological discomfort is often reported only as somatic or physical symptoms that are medically unexplained upon further evaluation. Different perceptions of what are both the causes and

Case #3

CW is a 19-year-old woman who was brought by her concerned parents to a behavioral health clinic for evaluation. She had recently been found by the police wandering aimlessly in her neighborhood late at night, having a conversation without anyone physically present, responding to internal stimuli, and laughing spontaneously without apparent reason. At first, CW's parents thought that their daughter had lost her soul, and consulted with local healers who could provide the ceremonial rituals to regain it. When her behavior did not improve and in fact worsened, CW was hospitalized for treatment shortly after being evaluated at the clinic.

Question

1. What cultural issues emerge in CW's case that may inform the possible diagnosis of a psychotic disorder such as schizophrenia?

Table 4-4 Elements of the Cultural Formulation Interview (CFI)

Questions	Guidance for the Interviewer
Cultural Definition of the Problem	
1. What brings you here today? How would *you* describe your problem?	Try to keep the focus on the individual's own conceptualization of the clinical presentation. Use the patient's own language in referring to the problem during the remainder of the interview.
2. How would you describe (your problem) to your family, friends, or others in your community?	This clarifies how the individual frames the clinical presentation for members of her or his social network.
3. What troubles you most about (your problem)?	This identifies how the individual prioritizes the impact of the clinical presentation.
Cultural Perceptions of Cause, Context, and Support	
4. Why do you think this has happened? What do you believe are the causes of (your problem)? For example, some people may think that their problems are due to bad things that have happened in their lives, a physical cause, a spiritual cause, or something else.	It is important to determine the meaning of the condition to the individual, which may be relevant to future adherence to the treatment plan.
5. What do others among your family, your friends, or others in your community think is causing (your problem)?	The perceptions of the social network may be different than that of the individual, and this may help determine whether the clinical presentation is at variance with the cultural norm.
6. Are there any kinds of support that make (your problem) better, such as from family, friends, or others?	The existence of support systems familiar to the individual may enhance resilience in the face of the clinical presentation.
7. Are there any kinds of stresses that make (your problem) worse, such as difficulties with money or within the family?	Knowledge of specific stressors or triggers that may exacerbate the presenting symptoms would be helpful.
8. What are the most important aspects of your background or identity?	Sometimes an individual's native language; ethnic, racial, or cultural community; place of origin; gender or gender expression; faith tradition; or sexual orientation may affect the nature and course of the clinical presentation.
9. Are there any aspects of your background or identity that make a difference to (your problem)?	This may identify issues specific to the individual that may promote clinical worsening as a result of discrimination due to migration status, race/ethnicity, sexual orientation, etc.
10. Are there any aspects of your background or identity that are causing other difficulties for you?	Probing for additional contexts in these areas can be useful (e.g., migration-related problems, conflict across generations, limitations of gender roles).

(continues)

Table 4-4 Elements of the Cultural Formulation Interview (CFI) (*continued*)

Questions	Guidance for the Interviewer
Cultural Factors Affecting Self-Coping and Past Help-Seeking	
11. Sometimes people have various ways of dealing with situations like (your problem). What have you done on your own to cope?	This helps the clinician to identify the existing internal resources of the individual.
12. Sometimes people seek help from many different sources, including different types of doctors, helpers, or healers. In the past, what kinds of treatment, help, advice, or healing have you sought for (your problem)? What types of help or treatment were most useful? What types were not useful?	Clarification of the individual's own experience and regard for assistance may inform the treatment plan.
13. Has anything prevented you from getting the help you need (e.g., money, insurance, work or family obligations, stigma or discrimination, lack of services that understand your native language or background)?	There are often numerous social barriers that prevent access to appropriate care.
Cultural Factors Affecting Current Help-Seeking	
14. What help do you think would be most useful to you at this time for (your problem)?	This clarifies the individual's current perceived needs and expectations of help.
15. Are there other kinds of help that your family, friends, or other people have suggested that would be helpful for you now?	This acknowledges that there may be influences by the individual's social network that may impact seeking help for managing clinical symptoms.
16. There are times that doctors and patients misunderstand each other because they come from different backgrounds or have different expectations. Have you been concerned about this, and is there anything that we can do to provide the care you need?	Information provided in response to this question may allow clinicians to address specific barriers to care or concerns about the clinic or the clinician–patient relationship.

Data from American Psychiatric Association. *Diagnostic and Statistical Manual of Mental Disorders*. 5th ed. (DSM-5). Arlington, VA: American Psychiatric Association; 2013.

manifestations of "illness" may also impede the development of an effective therapeutic plan. A reframing of what constitutes a disorder into what causes distress in an individual described in that person's own words may serve as a more useful starting point for assessment according to the DSM-5 Outline for Cultural Formulation. For someone from a family-based culture, enlisting the support and cooperation of family members might be an essential component of care once a plan is established. With respectful intentionality, consultations with a folk healer or an esteemed clergy/spiritual practitioner held in high regard by the individual may lead to a beneficial and collaborative approach to treatment.

Case #4

FD is a 24-year-old man who was born in a tropical country to an ethnic minority family that is extremely religious. The family immigrated to the United States when FD was a teenager. He had been gainfully employed as a taxi driver 7 days a week until he started to have trouble sleeping with complaints of hearing voices and having racing thoughts. He also began to feel more suspicious toward others, including members of his family, who he perceived as threatening him. In order to gain some relief, FD began to excessively drink alcohol to the point of being arrested for driving under the influence—which resulted in the loss of his driver's license and source of income. His mother blamed his problems on his not attending church on Sunday and not praying hard enough, and his unusual behavior was due to "not being right with God." FD attributed his hardship to someone in his homeland placing a curse on him.

Question

1. What cultural issues may come into play when assessing FD's case?

Summary

Assessments of mental health and behavior rely on the basic communication skills of careful listening and observation. Whether they are used for screening or diagnostic purposes, the clinician should understand that there can be great variability in the clinical presentation of any given psychiatric diagnosis among patients. There may also be significant overlap of symptoms across multiple diagnoses. Attention to documenting the actual manifestations of psychological distress as they appear in a specific individual is critical to the development of a rational therapeutic plan. The most commonly used tools to determine this are the clinical interview and the mental status examination; supplemental information may be obtained by the administration of self-rating questionnaires.

The ultimate goal of fully embracing cultural considerations during psychiatric assessment is to help reduce the barriers to a trusting therapeutic relationship between an individual and a clinician who may each hold different perspectives regarding mental health and treatment. Once an appropriate level of mutual trust has been achieved at baseline, the likelihood of effectively monitoring therapeutic outcomes going forward will be enhanced.

Review Questions

1. What is the primary clinician-administered assessment tool used in determining symptoms reflecting altered mental status or behavior that may require treatment?
2. What are the five general domains assessed in this tool?
3. Before this assessment is made, what needs to be performed once it has been determined that changes in mental status or behavior have occurred?
4. What are some self-assessment tools that a pharmacist might be able to assist a patient with in order to screen for referrals to a behavioral health specialist?

References

American Psychiatric Association. *Diagnostic and Statistical Manual of Mental Disorders*. 5th ed. (DSM-5). Arlington, VA: American Psychiatric Association; 2013.

American Psychiatric Association. Practice guideline for the psychiatric evaluation of adults, 2nd edition. *Am J Psychiatry*. 2006;163(6 Suppl):1–62.

Beck AT, Steer A. Internal consistencies of the original and revised Beck Depression Inventory. *J Clin Psychol*. 1984;40(6):1365–1367.

Chu J, Floyd R, Diep H, Pardo S, Goldblum P, Bongar B. A tool for the culturally competent assessment of suicide: The Cultural Assessment of Risk for Suicide (CARS) measure. *Psychological Assessment*, Vol 25(2), Jun 2013, 424–434. doi: 10.1037/a0031264

Chu JP, Goldblum P, Floyd R, Bongar B. A cultural theory and model of suicide. *Appl Prevent Psychol*. 2010;14:25–40.

DiPiro JT, Talbert RL, Yee GC, Matzke GR, Wells BG, Posey LM, eds. *Pharmacotherapy: A Pathophysiologic Approach*. 8th ed. New York: McGraw-Hill; 2011.

Snyderman D, Rovner BW. Mental status examination in primary care: A review. *Am Fam Physician*. 2009;80(8):809–814.

Spitzer RL, Williams JBW, Kroenke K, Linzer M, deGruy FV, Hahn SR, et al. Utility of a new procedure for diagnosing mental disorders in primary care: The PRIME-MD 1000 study. *JAMA*. 1994;272:1749–1756.

U.S. Department of Health and Human Services. Executive summary. In: *Mental Health: Culture, Race, and Ethnicity. A Supplement to Mental Health: A Report of the Surgeon General*. Rockville, MD: U.S. Department of Health and Human Services, Public Health Service, Office of the Surgeon General; 2001. Available at: http://www.ncbi.nlm.nih.gov/books/NBK44243/?report=printable. Accessed May 31, 2013.

Zung A. A self-rating depression scale. *Arch Gen Psychiatry*. 1965;12(1):63–70.

Chapter 5

Dermatological Assessment

Heather Fields, PharmD, MPH, BCACP
Carmita A. Coleman, PharmD, MAA

LEARNING OBJECTIVES

At the completion of this chapter, the reader should be able to

1. Determine appropriate questions to ask patients when performing a dermatological interview.
2. Explain the clinical presentation of common symptoms and diseases related to dermatology.
3. Explain how to correctly perform the physical assessment techniques related to dermatology.
4. List medications that can cause adverse effects or medical conditions affecting hair, skin, and nails.
5. Explain the clinical presentation of drug-induced disease processes.
6. Identify differences in clinical presentation of certain conditions in patients of various ethnic groups.

KEY TERMS

Acanthosis nigricans	Erythema	Pruritus
Comedones	Hyperpigmentation	Pseudofolliculitis barbae
Contact dermatitis	Keloids	Tinea
Eruptions	Lesions	Xerosis

Introduction

The pharmacist's ability to perform a dermatological assessment is a valuable skill in any practice setting. In community and clinical pharmacy settings, assessment of the skin, hair, and nails can help to identify dermatology disorders, adverse drug reactions, or drug allergies. This information can assist the pharmacist in making self-care recommendations, identifying a drug-related problem, or referring the patient to a physician. The dermatological assessment performed by a pharmacist is rather limited, and the extent to which these assessments can be performed may be dependent on the amount of privacy available at the practice location.

© antishock/Shutterstock, Inc.

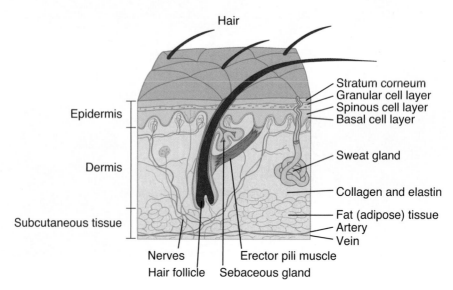

Hair

Epidermis

Dermis

Subcutaneous tissue

Stratum corneum
Granular cell layer
Spinous cell layer
Basal cell layer

Sweat gland

Collagen and elastin

Fat (adipose) tissue
Artery
Vein

Nerves   Erector pili muscle
Hair follicle   Sebaceous gland

FIGURE 5-1 Skin anatomy.

The skin is the body's largest organ. It is composed of three layers: the epidermis, dermis, and hypodermis (subcutaneous tissue) (**FIGURE 5-1**). The epidermis is the outermost protective layer, the dermis is the underlying layer composed of connective tissue, and the hypodermis is the deepest layer made of subcutaneous tissue. Sebaceous and sweat glands, keratinocytes, and melanocytes also contribute to the structural composition of the skin. Hair originates from follicles in the dermis, and there are two types of hair that exist on the human body. Vellus hair is short, fine, and nonpigmented, and covers most of the body on children and adults. Terminal hair is longer, thicker, and pigmented compared to vellus hair, and is stimulated by puberty (e.g., pubic hair). Nails are located on the dorsal surface of the hands and feet (**FIGURE 5-2**). They are made of a keratin matrix that comprises the nail plate. This plate is situated on top of the nail bed, which is supplied by a vascular network. Both hair and nails are skin appendages. This entire system serves as a barrier by inhibiting fluid loss and entrance of pathogens. Additional functions of the skin include regulating body temperature, preventing dehydration, and sensory activity. Due to the skin being the largest and outermost organ of the body, it is susceptible to many conditions.

The patient interview should include questions that will aid in identifying a possible cause of the dermatology disorder. For example, the interview should include questions regarding previous exposure to chemicals, plants, or animals, and recent changes in soaps, moisturizers, cosmetics, or laundry detergents. In addition, the pharmacist should ask about any recent exposure to people who may have a skin condition or recent infection. Lastly, along with reviewing the patient's medication history, the pharmacist should inquire about medication allergies, the use of new prescription or over-the-counter (OTC) medications, and the use of herbal products. Particular attention should be paid if the patient has recently or is currently taking medications that are known to cause dermatologic adverse effects and reactions.

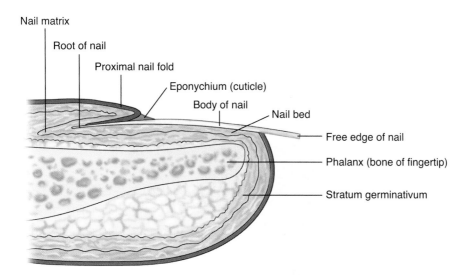

Nail matrix
Root of nail
Proximal nail fold
Eponychium (cuticle)
Body of nail
Nail bed
Free edge of nail
Phalanx (bone of fingertip)
Stratum germinativum

FIGURE 5-2 Nail anatomy.

The dermatology assessment involves both inspection and palpation of the skin, hair, and nails (**Table 5-1**). Palpation is to use hands when performing the physical examination. The pharmacist should use gloves when completing this portion of the assessment. Inspection involves visual observation of the skin. Due to the visibility of the skin, a physical exam can easily occur through clinical observation. Depending on the level of privacy, the pharmacist may have to view areas that are hidden by clothing or are inappropriate to show in semi-private examination areas. Sufficient lighting should also be available to conduct a proper exam (DiSimone, 2002). The assessment should identify skin, hair, and nail characteristics, including the presence of skin **lesions**. Lesions are any pathologic skin change or occurrence and may be primary (caused by a disease process or trauma) or secondary (occurs as a result of a primary lesion). When checking for skin lesions, note their location, quantity, size, shape (e.g., ring-shaped or linear), distribution (i.e., generalized over body or localized to one area), and pattern (i.e., grouped or diffuse). Also identify the color and pigmentation, surface features (i.e., smooth or rough), depth or elevation, and type of skin lesion present. **Table 5-2** describes different lesions that may be present on the skin.

Lesions:
A localized area of damage on an organ or tissue resulting from injury or disease. May be primary or secondary in origin. Primary lesions are caused by a disease process or trauma; secondary lesions occur as a result of primary lesions.

Table 5-1 Dermatology Examination Summary

	Inspection	Palpation
Skin	Color and pigmentation, odor, symmetry, uniformity, cleanliness, thickness, lesions	Moisture, temperature, texture, mobility, turgor, pain
Hair	Quantity, color, distribution	Texture
Nails	Color and pigmentation, shape, length, similarity, splitting, ridging, curvature	Thickness, texture, attachment to nail bed, pliability, pain, uniformity

Data from Bickley LS and Szilagyi P. The skin, hair, and nails. In: Bickley LS and Szilagyi P, eds. *Bates' Guide to Physical Examination and History Taking*. 10th ed. Philadelphia, PA: Lippincott Williams & Wilkins; 2009:163–190; Seidel HM, Ball JW, Dains JE, Benedict GW, eds. *Mosby's Guide to Physical Examination*. 6th ed. St. Louis, MO: Elsevier; 2006:169–229.

Table 5-2 Differentiation of Skin

Term	Type	Description	Example
		Superficial Lesions	
Macule	Primary	Circumscribed flat area with a change in skin color less than 1 cm in diameter	Freckles, flat mole, measles

© Manuela Krause/Stock

© robert lerich/Stock/Thinkstock

(continues)

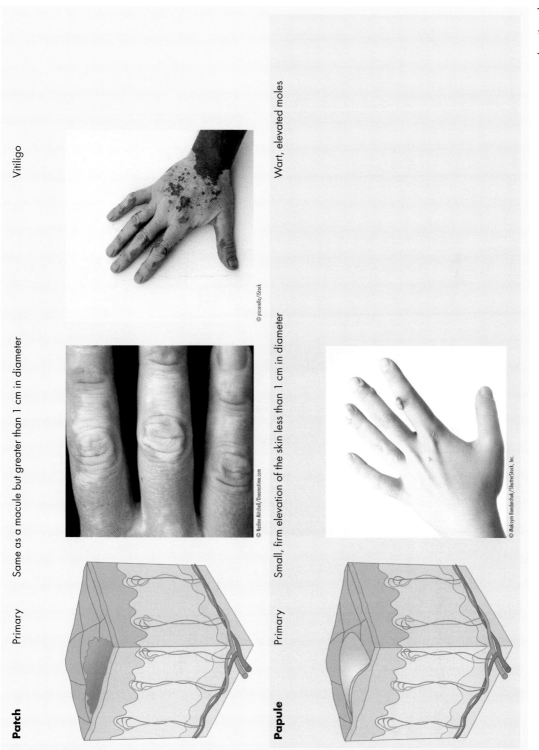

Patch

Primary

Same as a macule but greater than 1 cm in diameter

Vitiligo

© picareilly/iStock

© Nadine Mitchell/Dreamstime.com

Papule

Primary

Small, firm elevation of the skin less than 1 cm in diameter

Wart, elevated moles

© Maksym Bondarchuk/ShutterStock, Inc.

Table 5-2 Differentiation of Skin (continued)

Term	Type	Description			Example
Plaque	Primary	Solid, flatter, raised skin less than 1 cm in diameter			Psoriasis

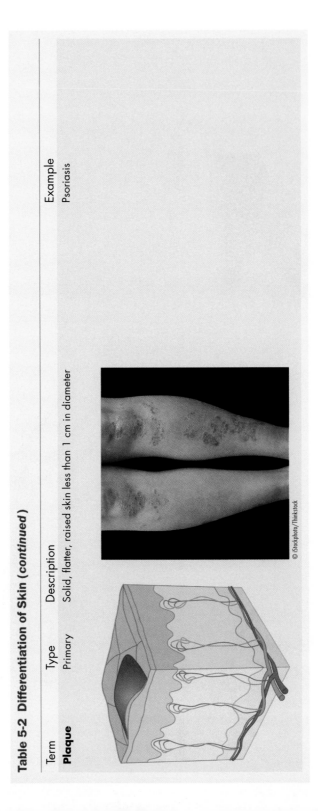

© iStockphoto/Thinkstock

(continues)

Wheal

Primary

Raised area of edema on the epidermis with a variable diameter

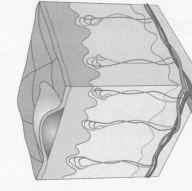

© Dr. P. Marazzi/Science Source

Insect bites, allergic reactions, urticaria

Vesicle

Primary

Raised area of skin filled with clear fluid less than 1 cm in diameter

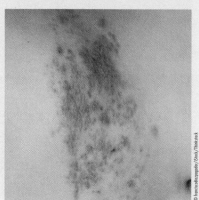

© franciscodiazpagador/iStock/Thinkstock

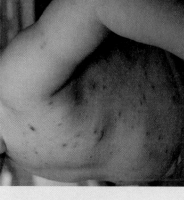

© jar gennall/iStock/Thinkstock

Varicella (chickenpox), herpes zoster (shingles)

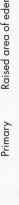

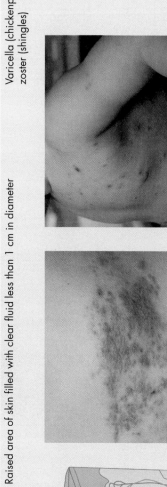

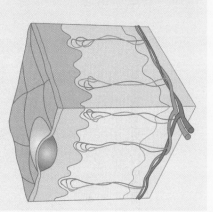

Table 5-2 Differentiation of Skin (*continued*)

Term	Type	Description			Example
Bulla	Primary	Vesicle greater than 1 cm in diameter			Blister

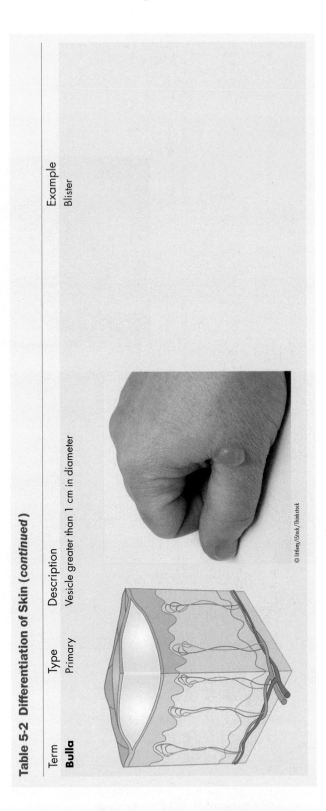

© Ittiteny/iStock/Thinkstock

(continues)

Pustule

Primary

A small, raised area of the epidermis filled with pus

Impetigo, acne

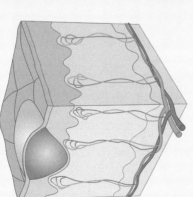

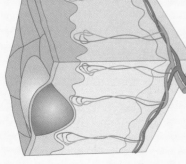

© olovs/ShutterStock, Inc.

Scale

Secondary

An accumulation of loose, desquamated skin cells

Dry skin, flaking of skin following a drug reaction

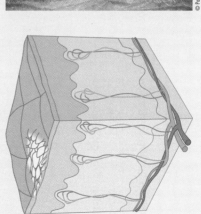

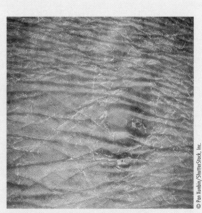

© Pan Xunbin/ShutterStock, Inc.

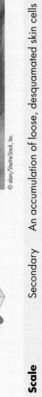

Table 5-2 Differentiation of Skin (continued)

Term	Type	Description	Example
Lichenification	Secondary	Thickening of the epidermis due to chronic irritation, rubbing, or itching	Chronic dermatitis

(continues)

Crust (scab)

Secondary   Dried exudates, from either serum, blood, pus, or a combination

Scab on abrasion, eczema

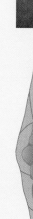

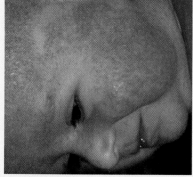

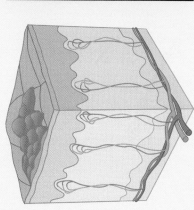

© SPL/Custom Medical Stock Photo

Deep Lesions

Tumor

Primary   Solid, raised mass less than
1 cm in diameter that extends into deeper layers of the skin

Neoplasm, lipoma

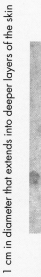

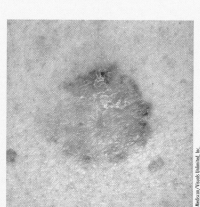

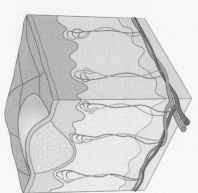

© Medscan/Visuals Unlimited, Inc.

Table 5-2 Differentiation of Skin (*continued*)

Term	Type	Description	Example
Nodule	Primary	Solid, raised skin less than 1 cm in diameter that extends into the deeper skin layers	Lipoma

© Dr. P. Marazzi/Science Source

(continues)

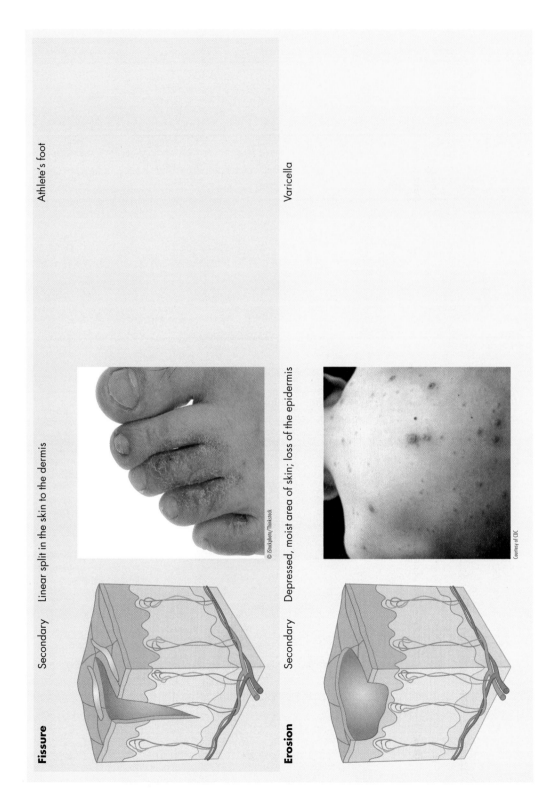

Fissure   Secondary   Linear split in the skin to the dermis   Athlete's foot

© iStockphoto/Thinkstock

Erosion   Secondary   Depressed, moist area of skin; loss of the epidermis   Varicella

Courtesy of CDC

Table 5-2 Differentiation of Skin (*continued*)

Term	Type	Description		Example
Ulcer	Secondary	Loss of epidermis and dermis	 Courtesy of Dr. Steve Kraus/CDC	Stasis ulcers

Both Superficial and Deep Lesions

Cyst   Primary   Raised cavity in deeper skin layers filled with liquid or semi-solid material

Cystic acne

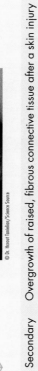

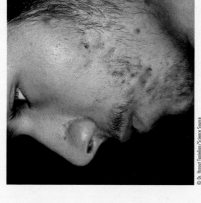

© Dr. Harout Tanielian/Science Source

Keloid   Secondary   Overgrowth of raised, fibrous connective tissue after a skin injury

Keloid formation following surgery

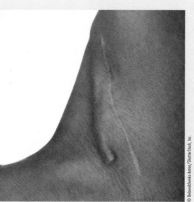

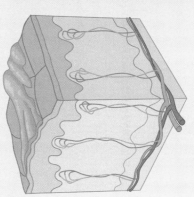

© Belovodchenko Antoy/ShutterStock, Inc.

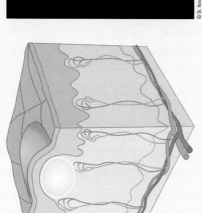

(continues)

Table 5-2 Differentiation of Skin (*continued*)

Term	Type	Description	Example
Scar	Secondary	Thin to thick area of fibrous tissue that replaced damaged skin	Healed wound after injury

© Dr. P. Marazzi/Science Source

Atrophy

Secondary

Thinning or absence of the skin surface

Aged skin

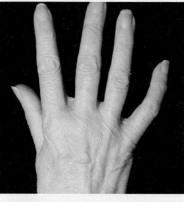

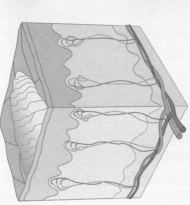

© Ralph Hutchings/Visuals Unlimited, Inc.

Data from Seidel HM, Ball JW, Dains JE, Benedict GW, eds. *Mosby's Guide to Physical Examination.* 6th ed. St. Louis, MO: Elsevier; 2006:169–229.

Clinical Presentation of Disease Processes Related to Skin, Hair, and Nails

Acne

Comedones:
Noninflammatory skin lesion that is the primary sign of acne. It is composed of the dilated hair follicle, skin debris, bacteria, and sebum. May be open or closed. Open comedones are called blackheads; closed comedones are referred to as whiteheads.

Acne is the most common dermatological skin condition in the United States. It is most prevalent in adolescents; however, it can affect adults. Acne is characterized by the presence of noninflammatory (**comedones;** FIGURE 5-3) and inflammatory (papule, pustule, nodule, or cyst; FIGURES 5-4 and 5-5) lesions. Noninflammatory comedone lesions related to acne are referred to as blackheads or whiteheads. Blackheads (open comedones) are dark or yellow in appearance. Whiteheads (closed comedones) are white in appearance, and can sometimes be associated with inflammatory nodules or cysts.

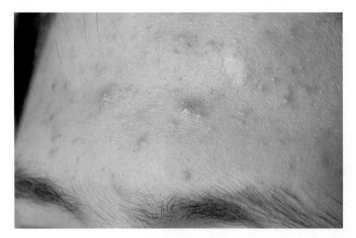

FIGURE 5-3 Comedonal acne on forehead.
© olavs/Shutterstock, Inc.

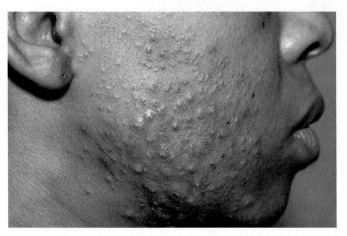

FIGURE 5-4 Inflammatory acne lesions causing hyperpigmentation.
© John F. Wilson/Science Source

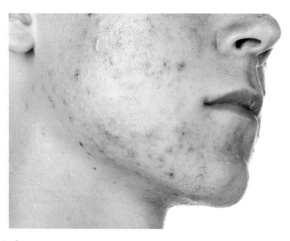

FIGURE 5-5 Severe cystic acne.
© Suzanne Tucker/ShutterStock, Inc.

Generally acne is categorized as either mild, moderate, or severe (**Table 5-3**). Mild acne may be treated with self-care measures and OTC products. Patients with moderate or severe acne should be referred to their primary care provider for further assessment and treatment (Quairoli, 2009).

The Patient Interview

When interviewing a patient about acne, it is important to determine the onset and frequency of acne outbreaks. Precipitating factors can cause acne outbreaks; therefore, questions regarding the temporal relationship of an acne outbreak and situations such as stress and menses (in women) should be assessed. In addition, the patient should be interviewed about wearing occlusive clothing, use of cosmetics, and excessive sweat in the areas affected by the acne. The pharmacist should also inquire about any products the patient has used

Table 5-3 Sample IGA Scale for Acne Vulgaris

Grade	Description
0	Clear skin with no inflammatory or noninflammatory lesions
1	Almost clear; rare noninflammatory lesions with no more than one small inflammatory lesion
2	Mild severity; greater than Grade 1; some noninflammatory lesions with no more than a few inflammatory lesions (papules/pustules only, no nodular lesions)
3	Moderate severity; greater than Grade 2; up to many noninflammatory lesions and may have some inflammatory lesions, but no more than one small nodular lesion
4*	Severe; greater than Grade 3; up to many noninflammatory and inflammatory lesions, but no more than a few nodular lesions

* The Case Report Forms for acne studies can allow for reporting by investigators of lesion worsening beyond Grade 4 with treatment. It is recommended that enrollment of acne vulgaris patients not include patients with nodulocystic acne. Patients who worsen beyond Grade 4 are to be described in the safety evaluation.

Reproduced from Center for Drug Evaluation and Research (CDER). *Guidance for Industry Acne Vulgaris: Developing Drugs for Treatment.* U.S. Department of Health and Human Services and Food and Drug Administration, 2005.

to try to relieve or improve the acne. Lastly, a complete history of prescription and OTC medications should be obtained to determine if the patient has used any medications that are known to cause drug-induced acne. Patients who have failed OTC acne treatment products after 6 weeks of use should be referred to a medical provider (Quairoli, 2009).

The Physical Exam

The physical assessment begins with observation of the acne lesions in the affected areas. The pharmacists should assess the location and distribution of the lesions on the body, as well as the amount and types of lesions present to determine the severity of acne present (Sibbald, 2011).

Xerosis (Dry Skin)

Xerosis:
Abnormal dryness of a body part or tissue, especially of the skin, eye, or mucous membranes.

Xerosis, also known as dry skin, is caused by decreased water and oil content of the stratum corneum in the epidermis layer of the skin. It is the most common cause of **pruritus**, commonly referred to as itching. It can occur in individuals of all ages but largely affects older adults. Generally, dry skin can be managed through self-care measures with improved bathing practices and use of emollients or antipruritic agents. However, if skin dryness persists after 7 days of treatment, the patient should be referred for medical attention (Scott, 2009).

The Patient Interview

Pruritus:
Itching sensation.

When assessing a patient with dry skin, it is important to ask about bathing habits. Bathing frequently or for a prolonged period of time, bathing in hot water, or excessive use of harsh soaps and cleansers can contribute to dry skin. Also, decreased water intake can worsen skin hydration, so asking the patient about daily water consumption is helpful. Environmental factors, such as cold weather, low humidity, and high wind velocity, can contribute to dry skin because these can cause moisture loss in skin. Therefore, questions about environmental exposure should be included in the interview. Health conditions and medications that contribute to dry skin should be reviewed as well (Scott, 2009).

The Physical Exam

The physical examination for dry skin involves inspection of the affected area to determine the presence of skin roughness, flaking, and inflammation (**FIGURE 5-6**). Dry skin

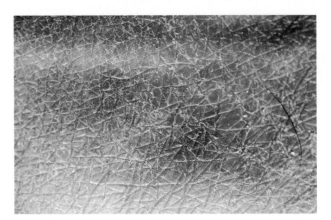

FIGURE 5-6 Xerosis (dry skin).
© Pan Xunbin/ShutterStock

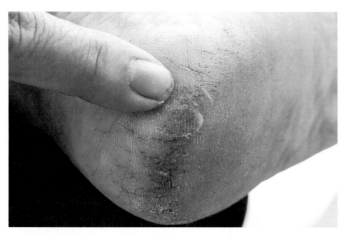

FIGURE 5-7 Dry, cracked skin on the heel of a foot.
© Amawasri/iStock/Thinkstock

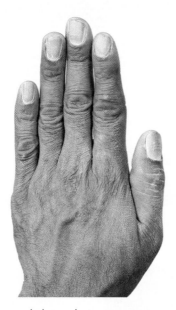

FIGURE 5-8 Dry, "ashy" skin on a dark complexion.
© itanistock/Alamy

can also present with a scaly, fish-like, or cracked appearance (**FIGURE 5-7**) with loss of flexibility (Scott, 2009). In people of color, dry skin may appear as a pale, gray, or whitish color, referred to as ashy (**FIGURE 5-8**). Dry skin is often located on the arms and legs, but can occur in any area of the body. Patients with skin that appears to be infected or oozing fluid should be referred to the primary care provider for further assessment.

Contact Dermatitis

Contact dermatitis is an acute inflammatory condition of the skin caused by an external substance. This condition commonly presents with red, burning, and pruritic skin.

Contact dermatitis: Acute inflammatory condition of the skin caused by an external substance. May be categorized as irritant or allergic. Irritant contact dermatitis is generally caused by exposure to a chemical or irritant that results in skin damage. Allergic contact dermatitis is triggered by an immune response from an allergen.

It is categorized as irritant or allergic contact dermatitis and can be acute or chronic in nature. Acute contact dermatitis results from a single large exposure or a few exposures to a potent substance; in contrast, repetitive exposure to weaker irritants may lead to a chronic condition. Irritant contact dermatitis (ICD) accounts for 80–90% of contact dermatitis cases (Newton, 2014). ICD is generally caused by a chemical or an agent that results in skin damage. The severity of ICD is dependent upon the quantity and concentration of the irritant exposure, the duration of contact with the irritant, and the condition of the skin. Common irritants include chemicals, solvents, and water. Symptoms can manifest within a few minutes for a single exposure to a few days or weeks for multiple exposures. Conversely, allergic contact dermatitis (ACD) is due to a hypersensitivity reaction from an allergen. An immunologic response usually occurs 24–72 hours after re-exposure to the causative substance. Common causes of ACD include poison ivy (**FIGURE 5-9**), poison oak, and poison sumac, all of which are triggered by exposure to the substance urushiol, which is found in the plants' leaves. Metal, such as nickel (**FIGURE 5-10**), and

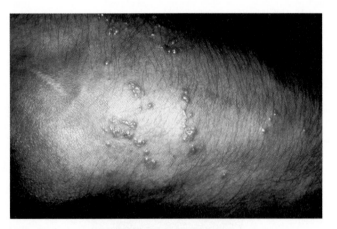

FIGURE 5-9 Allergic contact dermatitis from poison ivy.
Courtesy of the Center for Disease Control

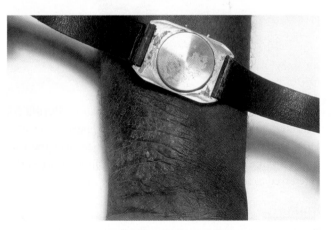

FIGURE 5-10 African American with allergic contact dermatitis from nickel in watchband.
© Medical-on-Line/Alamy

Table 5-4 Differentiation of Allergic and Irritant Contact Dermatitis

Symptom or Characteristic	Irritant Contact Dermatitis	Allergic Contact Dermatitis
Itching	Yes, later	Yes, early
Stinging, burning	Early	Late or not at all
Erythema	Yes	Yes
Vesicles, bullae	Rarely or no	Yes
Papules	Rarely or no	Yes
Dermal edema	Yes	Yes
Delayed reaction to exposure	Minutes to hours	Days, slower reaction
Appearance of symptoms in relation to exposure	Single or multiple exposures	Delayed
Causative substances	Water, urine, flour, detergents, hand sanitizers, soap, alkalis, acids, solvents, salts, surfactants, oxidizers	Low-molecular-weight and lipid-soluble substances, fragrances, nickel, latex, benzocaine, neomycin, leather
Substance concentration at exposure	Important	Less important
Mechanism of reaction	Direct tissue damage	Immunologic reaction
Location	Hands, wrist, forearms, diaper area	Anywhere on the body that comes in contact with antigen
Presentation	No clear margin	Clear margins based on contact of offending substance

Data from Plake KS, Darbishire PL. Contact dermatitis. In: Berardi RR, Ferreri SP, Hume AL, et al., eds. *Handbook of Nonprescription Drugs: An Interactive Approach to Self-Care*. 17th ed. Washington, DC: American Pharmacists Association; 2009:657–673.

latex also can cause ACD. Further differences between ICD and ACD are outlined in **Table 5-4**. Contact dermatitis generally resolves without any treatment in 7–21 days after removing the offending agent.

The Patient Interview

Identifying the underlying cause or ruling out underlying causes constitutes a significant portion of the patient interview. The interview should include questions aimed at determining what substance the patient has been exposed to and the temporal relationship to the onset of symptoms. The pharmacist should determine if the reaction is new or reoccurring. If it has occurred in the past, asking about what triggered the previous reaction may help to identify or confirm the offending agent that has caused the reaction. In addition to questioning about use of new soaps, lotions, moisturizers, and laundry detergents, the pharmacist should also inquire about occupational and environmental exposures. Furthermore, a history of medication and environmental allergies should be obtained.

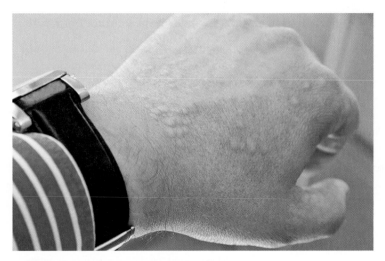

FIGURE 5-11 Irritant contact dermatitis on hand.
© Juergen Faelchle/Shutterstock, Inc.

If the patient has symptoms that are intolerable or limit completing normal daily activities, then referral to a primary care provider is acceptable.

The Physical Exam

The physical exam for both ICD and ACD involves visual inspection of the affected area. Contact dermatitis typically presents as a red rash (**FIGURE 5-11**), and the patient may complain of itching or pain. Symptoms vary depending on the type of contact dermatitis present, which is detailed in Table 5-4. The pharmacist should also take note of the size and location of the area affected by the rash. If the rash covers a large portion of the body, including the eyes, or appears to be infected, then the patient should be referred for treatment to the primary care provider.

Case #1

WG is a 29-year-old man who presents to the pharmacy with red, irritated hands occurring for the past week. His hands appear to be dry with scaly fissures. He states his hands are also itchy with minor pain. He does not have any vesicles, bullae, or signs of infection. No other areas of his body are affected and he has not experienced these symptoms before. He states he recently began a new job as a construction worker. Upon further questioning he tells you his hands are in repeated contact with wet concrete and solvents. He has asthma and takes albuterol prn.

Questions
1. What dermatological disorder is WG's complaint consistent with? Why?
2. Would you categorize WG's symptoms as irritant or allergic contact dermatitis? Why?
3. Is WG's condition chronic or acute? Why?
4. What additional questions can you ask this patient to differentiate between ICD and ACD?

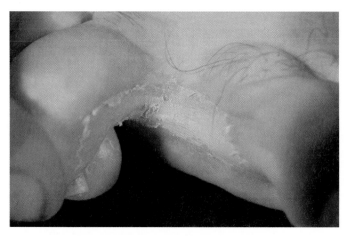

FIGURE 5-12 Tinea Pedis.
Courtesy of Dr. Lucille K. Georg/CDC

Fungal Infections

Fungal infections caused by dermatophytes are referred to as **tinea**, and are the most common fungal infection in humans. Also known as ringworm for their ring-shaped appearance, tinea infections are termed according to the location of the body affected. Fungal infections of the body, foot (athlete's foot; **FIGURE 5-12**), and groin (jock itch) can be treated with self-care measures such as OTC antifungal products; however, patients presenting with fungal infections of the scalp (**FIGURE 5-13**) or nails, or an infection

Tinea:
Fungal infection commonly caused by the *Dermatophyte* species.

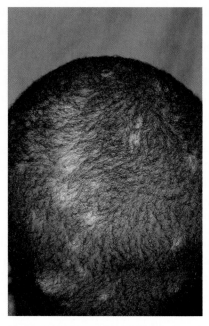

FIGURE 5-13 Tinea capitis in an African American child.
© Dr. Ken Greer/Visuals Unlimited, Inc.

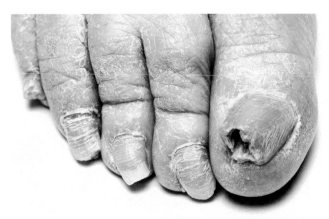

FIGURE 5-14 Onchyomycosis.
© lekcej/ShutterStock

caused by *Candida*, should be referred to the primary care provider. Also, patients presenting with severe symptoms, diabetes, or an immunocompromised condition should be referred for medical treatment.

The Patient Interview

The interview should determine the patient's onset of symptoms and identify any exposure to risk factors for fungal infections. Information regarding recent contact with people infected with a fungal infection, exposure to animals, and exposure to fungus in the environment should be obtained. Environments that are warm, humid, and moist create an atmosphere for fungus to grow, so moist areas of the body due to sweating may provide a favorable atmosphere for fungus to grow. Therefore, questioning the patient about hygiene, bathing practices, or exercising may help identify the underlying cause of the infection.

Nail fungal infections are called onychomycosis (**FIGURE 5-14**). Patients with this condition should be asked about nail injury, use of nail salons (including acrylic nails), history of nail disease, and overall nail hygiene practices because these are risk factors for nail fungal infections. Patients who have compromised immune systems or patients on medications that can suppress the immune system are at increased risk of developing fungal infections, so a thorough review of their past medical conditions and medication history is important. Lastly, the pharmacist should inquire about whether the patient has tried to treat the infection, and if so, what therapy was used.

The Physical Exam

Depending on the location of the rash, performing a physical examination of the affected area may be excluded. For patients presenting with a rash that can be easily viewed by the pharmacist, a physical exam consisting of inspection should occur. Inspection should identify the location of the rash and lesion characteristics. The pharmacist should also determine if malodor, scaling, inflammation, and fissures are present in the affected area. It is recommended that the pharmacist avoid touching the affected skin without gloves because fungal infections can be transmitted through skin contact.

Table 5-5 Differentiation of Tinea Skin Infections

Type	Signs	Symptoms
Tinea pedis (foot)	Erythema, scaling, erosion, cracks and fissures, malodor, ulcerations, vesicles, wet and soggy appearance	Pruritus, stinging
Tinea corporis (body)	Erythema, scales, circular and hyperpigmented plaques, vesicles, pustules	Pruritus
Tinea cruris (groin)	Erythema; bilateral, circular, and hyperpigmented plaques; scaling	Pruritus and pain
Tinea capitis (scalp)	Erythema, scaly patch on scalp, inflammation, plaques, pustules, hair loss with a gray patch or black dot where hair shaft is broken off at the scalp	Pain and tenderness
Tinea unguium (nail)	Opaque, thick, yellow, rough, brittle nails; separation from nail bed	Generally no pain or symptoms

Data from Goeser AL. Skin, hair, and nails. In: Jones RM, Rospond RM, eds. *Patient Assessment in Pharmacy Practice.* 2nd ed. Baltimore, MD: Lippincott Williams & Wilkins; 2009:118–140; Newton GD, Popovich NG. Fungal skin infections. In: Berardi RR, Ferreri SP, Hume AL, et al., eds. *Handbook of Nonprescription Drugs: An Interactive Approach to Self-Care.* 17th ed. Washington, DC: American Pharmacists Association; 2009:775–789.

Examination for onychomycosis involves inspecting the affected nails for changes in color and texture. A visual inspection of the nails, preferably clean and without nail polish, should occur. Affected nails appear thick, opaque, and brittle, and may appear separated from the nail bed. Signs and symptoms of fungal skin infections can vary depending on the region affected and are described in **Table 5-5**.

Burns

Burns are skin injuries caused by external sources. These sources are classified as thermal, ultraviolet (UV) radiation, electrical, and chemical. Burn wounds can occur through skin contact, ingestion, or inhalation. Thermal is the most common type of burn and is the result of contact with hot liquids, vapors, flames, or hot objects. Hot objects causing thermal burns include metal, plastic, and glass items, such as pots and pans, stove/oven, curling and clothing irons, and heaters. Scalding burns are caused by contact with hot liquids or gases, for instance, hot beverages, hot cooking oil, steam, and high-temperature bathing water. Other thermal burns can occur through the inhalation of steam or smoke.

Sunburn is an acute condition that results from a skin area being overexposed to UV radiation (**FIGURE 5-15**). The source of UV radiation can be natural (i.e., sunlight) or artificial (i.e., tanning beds or radiation therapy). Individuals with fair skin complexions are at greater risk for developing sunburns, but they can be prevented through use of sunscreen and protective clothing. Chronic sun exposure can lead to skin cancer; **hyperpigmentation**, also known as darkening of the skin; and photoaging (sun-induced aging skin characteristics).

Hyperpigmentation: Unusual darkened area of the skin or nails.

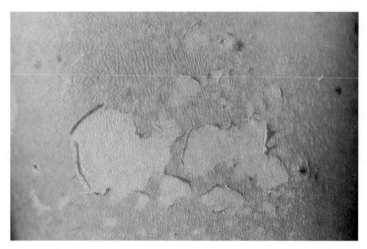

FIGURE 5-15 Peeling skin from sunburn.
© sezer66/iStock/Thinkstock

Chemical burns are from exposure to strong acids or alkalis, and can occur through skin contact or ingestion. These burns can worsen over time as the substance accumulates in skin and body tissue. The chemical will continue to cause damage until it is completely removed from the skin or neutralized. Electrical burns are caused by exposure to high-voltage electrical currents. These are considered thermal burns because the electrical current produces high-temperature heat. Lighting, electrical outlets, and extension cords are sources of electrical burns.

Burns are categorized by the depth of skin injury and the presentation of symptoms associated with the wound (**FIGURE 5-16**). Burn depths are classified from first-degree (superficial) to fourth-degree (extensive tissue damage) (**Table 5-6**). Minor burns can be treated with self-care measures, such as cool compresses, OTC antibiotics, antiseptics,

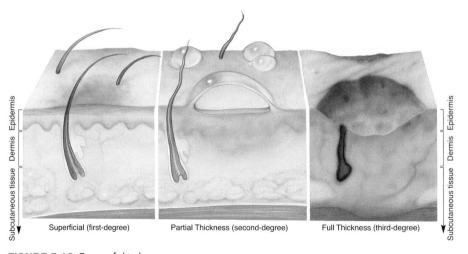

FIGURE 5-16 Types of skin burns.

Table 5-6 Classification of Burn Depth Injury

Type	Skin Layers Involved	Clinical Presentation	Healing Time	Examples
First-degree	Epidermis only	Erythema; mild to moderate pain; no skin breakage, blistering, or scarring	3 to 6 days	Minor sunburn, flash burn
Second-degree (partial-thickness)	Epidermis and superficial dermis	Blistering, erythema, moist, flexible, swelling, blanching with pressure, intense pain and tenderness (FIGURES 5-17 and 5-18)	1 to 3 weeks, typically without scarring	Severe sunburn, scalding liquid, brief contact with a hot object
Second-degree (deep-thickness)	Epidermis and dermis	White and red areas, dry, waxy, less flexible, decreased sensation and pain	Up to 6 weeks	Hot cooking oil, chemicals, flames
Third-degree	All epidermis, dermis, some subcutaneous fat; dermis appendages destroyed	White, tan, or red; dry, leathery; possible visible blood vessels; loss of pain and sensation (FIGURE 5-19)	Months to indefinite; excision, skin grafting; severe scarring	Flames, electricity, chemicals, extended exposure to hot objects
Fourth-degree	Extension of third-degree including muscle, tendon, and bone	Black, charred; skin necrosis; no pain or sensation	Indefinite; possible amputation or death	Prolonged exposure to third-degree causes

Reproduced with permission from EB Medicine, publisher of Emergency Medicine Practice, from: Adam J. Singer. Thermal burns: rapid assessment and treatment. Emergency Medicine Practice. 2000;2(9):1–20. www.ebmedicine.net.

and pain-relieving products. Patients presenting with moderate or severe burns, burns covering crucial areas, or comorbid conditions should seek urgent medical attention (Table 5-7).

The Patient Interview

When interviewing a patient with a burn wound, it is important to identify the source of the injury and the time the injury occurred. Inhalation, ingestion, electrical, and chemical burns have the ability to penetrate deeper tissues without being easily visible; therefore,

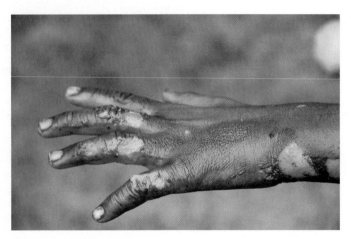

FIGURE 5-17 Deep partial-thickness burn.
© Naiyyer/ShutterStock

patients experiencing these types of burns need to seek medical attention immediately. In addition, the pharmacist should ask the patient about the time frame when the burn happened. This is important information because the severity of a burn can worsen 24–48 hours after the injury; therefore, reevaluation of the wound is necessary within the first few days. Also, obtaining the patient's past medical and medication history can help identify if the patient is at risk for complications. Any patient presenting with sunburn should be asked about their medications because photosensitivity reactions (discussed in the section Clinical Presentation of Drug-Induced Processes) appear as sunburns.

The Physical Exam

Physical assessment of a burn involves visual inspection of the depth, size, and location of the wound to determine its severity (Table 5-7). The depth of the burn depends on the degree of skin damage, as previously discussed. Furthermore, the clinical presentation

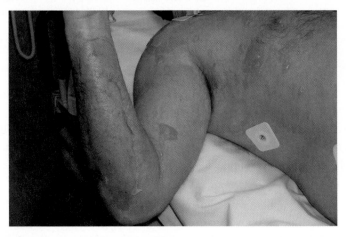

FIGURE 5-18 Second-degree burn with blistering.
© E.M. Singletary, M.D. Used with permission.

Table 5-7 Burn Severity Classification

Type of Burn	Children and Elderly	Adult
Minor	• Less than 10% BSA • Third- or fourth-degree covering less than 2% TBSA	• Less than 15% BSA • Third- or fourth-degree covering less than 2% BSA
Moderate	• 10–20% BSA • Third- or fourth-degree covering less than 10% BSA—not involving crucial areas*	• 15–25% TBSA • Third- or fourth-degree covering less than 10% BSA—not involving crucial areas*
Severe	• Greater than 20% BSA • Third- or fourth-degree covering less than 10% BSA • Crucial burn areas* • Complicated burns**	• Greater than 25% BSA • Third- or fourth-degree covering less than 10% BSA • Crucial burn areas* • Complicated burns**

BSA, body surface area; TBSA, total body surface area

*Crucial areas involve the face, perineum, eyes, and ears.

**Burns at risk for complications include electrical and inhalation burns, injuries involving major trauma, those involving infants or the elderly, and burns on patients with preexisting medical conditions.

Reproduced with permission from EB Medicine, publisher of Emergency Medicine Practice, from: Adam J. Singer. Thermal burns: rapid assessment and treatment. Emergency Medicine Practice. 2000;2(9):1–20. www.ebmedicine.net.

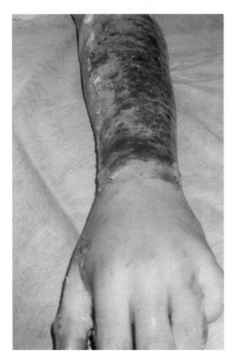

FIGURE 5-19 Third-degree burn.
© B. Slaven/Custom Medical Stock Photo

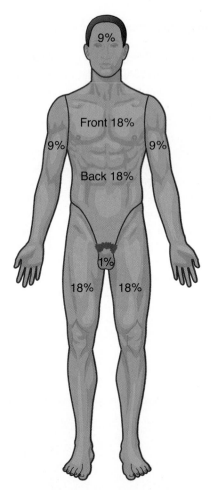

FIGURE 5-20 Rule of nines to estimate the amount of body surface area affected by a burn wound.

of symptoms, such as pain, blisters, swelling, and erythema, can help infer the depth of the wound. The size of a burn is determined by the percentage of body surface area (BSA) affected. The "rule of nines" is used as a guide to estimate how much BSA is involved with the burn wound (**FIGURE 5-20**). This rule applies only to second- and third-degree burns, and uses the size of a patient's palm to estimate approximately 1% of BSA. It is important to note that this rule is accurate in adults but not children. Also check to see if the patient is having respiratory distress or altered mental status because these symptoms may suggest loss of oxygen from an inhalation burn.

Moles and Skin Growths

Moles are skin lesions that can appear on any area of the body. Most moles are benign and asymptomatic; however, some moles can be a precursor in the development of skin cancer. Proper assessment of the appearance of the mole is important, because early detection of abnormalities of the mole can lead to prevention and early treatment for skin cancers.

The Patient Interview

A patient may approach the pharmacist about a mole if he or she feels it is cosmetically undesirable or has a concern about skin cancer. In other situations, the pharmacist may happen to notice a mole that looks abnormal and bring it to the attention of the patient. Regardless of the approach used for the patient interview, obtaining information about the patient's exposure to sunlight and ultraviolet radiation and their use of sun protection measures is important. The pharmacist should also ask about tanning practices, radiation exposure, and if the patient has ever experienced severe sunburns that involved blistering.

The Physical Exam

The visual inspection of moles is essential in determining if a patient should seek medical attention because cancerous moles generally differ in appearance from noncancerous moles (**FIGURE 5-21**). The ABCDE rule is a common screening tool used to examine moles or new skin spots for skin cancer (American Association of Dermatology, 2013) (**Table 5-8**). Early detection of skin cancer greatly improves prognosis. If a mole has any of the characteristics of ABCDE or if a mole is new, growing, bleeding, or itching then the patient should be referred to a dermatologist (National Cancer Institute, 2013).

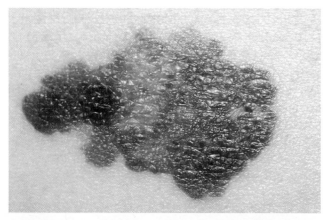

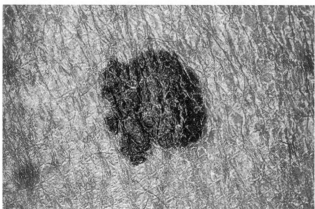

FIGURE 5-21 Melanoma.

(Top) Courtesy of the National Cancer Institute. (Bottom) Courtesy of Carl Washington and Mona Saraiya/CDC

Table 5-8 ABCDE Rule of Skin Cancer

Asymmetry	One half is different than the other half
Border	An irregular or poorly defined border
Color	Varies from one area to another
Diameter	Change in size, usually greater than 6 mm
Evolution	Change in size, shape, or color

Modified from National Cancer Institute. Symptoms of Melanoma. Available at: http://www.cancer.gov/cancertopics/wyntk/skin/page6.

Alopecia

Alopecia, also known as hair loss, affects both women (**FIGURE 5-22**) and men (**FIGURE 5-23**). It is normal for people to shed hair daily; however, when noticeable bald patches or hair thinning occurs, it can become problematic. Alopecia can be classified as nonscarring and scarring. Scarring alopecia is associated with scar formation and can lead to permanent loss and destruction of the hair follicle. Discoid lupus erythematous, syphilis, tinea capitis, and lichen planus are conditions that may be related to scarring alopecia.

Nonscarring is the most prevalent form of alopecia and is not related to permanent hair loss. The most common cause of nonscarring alopecia is pattern hair loss, which can be hereditary; however, there are other causes of hair loss such as stress, illness, hormonal disturbances, poor hair care practices, and chemotherapy (**Table 5-9**). If the patient is using hair care products or grooming practices that cause hair loss, then the patient should be advised to discontinue them. Typically once the causative factor is resolved the hair will begin to grow back in several weeks to months. Hereditary alopecia can be treated with OTC minoxidil. If therapy fails after 4 months of treatment or if the patient is experiencing hair loss for any other reason, then refer him or her to a dermatologist.

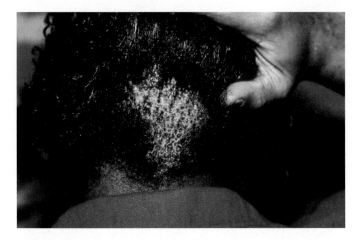

FIGURE 5-22 African American woman with alopecia.
© Z038/Custom Medical Stock Photo

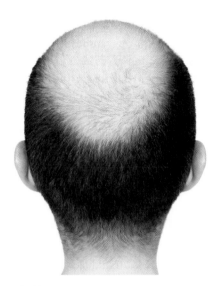

FIGURE 5-23 Male pattern baldness.
© Ilya Andriyanov/ShutterStock, Inc.

The Patient Interview

The patient interview should address not only the medical and medication history of the patient with alopecia, but also regular grooming practices that may increase the chances of hair loss. Using chemicals, high heat devices, rubber bands, and improper hair washing techniques can lead to hair damage and breakage. In addition, questioning the patient in regard to whether the hair loss occurred gradually over time or in a more accelerated manner is also helpful.

Table 5-9 Examples of Causes of Hair Loss

Anabolic steroids
Anemia
Chemotherapy
Hair accessories
Hair chemicals
Hormonal changes (pregnancy, menopause)
Hyperthyroidism
Hypothyroidism
Illness
Oral contraceptives
Poor nutrition

Data from Berry TM. Hair loss. In: Berardi RR, Ferreri SP, Hume AL, et al., eds. *Handbook of Nonprescription Drugs: An Interactive Approach to Self-Care.* 17th ed. Washington, DC: American Pharmacists Association; 2009:811–821; Valeyrie-Allanore L, Sassolas B, Roujeau JC. Drug-induced skin, nail, and hair disorders. *Drug Saf.* 2007;30:1011–1030. Available at: http://www.pharmpress.com/files/docs/ADRe2Ch05.pdf. Accessed March 20, 2013; Lee A, Thomson J. Drug-induced skin reactions. In: *Adverse Drug Reactions.* 2nd ed. London, England: Pharmaceutical Press; 2006:125–154. Available at: http://www.pharmpress.com/files/docs/ADRe2Ch05.pdf. Accessed March 20, 2013.

The Physical Exam

The physical examination for alopecia involves inspection of the scalp, eyelashes, eyebrows, and overall body for hair loss. Inspection of the nails is also important, because hair loss may coincide with nail abnormalities. When inspecting the area affected by hair loss, the pharmacist should determine if there is a pattern of hair loss and if any inflammation is present. Although a dermatologist or primary care provider may perform a "hair-pull test," in which the healthcare provider grasps and firmly pulls 40–60 hairs away from the scalp to assess the severity of hair loss, this test would not be appropriate for a pharmacist to perform. Rather, as a part of the patient interview, the pharmacist may ask the patient about how much hair is lost when combing or brushing the hair.

Clinical Presentation of Drug-Induced Processes

Eruptions:
Breaking out of a rash on the skin or a mucous membrane. A drug eruption is an adverse reaction to drug therapy.

Drug-induced skin **eruptions**, or skin breakouts with a rash, are a common problem related to drug therapy. Numerous medications can induce skin reactions. Although most reactions are not serious, some may cause severe, life-threatening complications. Skin eruptions generally present with some type of lesion, but mucus membranes and systemic multi-organ involvement also can occur. Drug-induced cutaneous (skin) conditions may be caused by both immune (i.e., lupus or human immunodeficiency virus [HIV]) and nonimmune processes. Most skin reactions are acute in nature and resolve within days to weeks, but some have chronic, long-lasting effects. In addition, medication-related skin reactions may induce or exacerbate a current or previous skin disorder. Secondary pigmentation changes associated with these eruptions are a result of increased melanin production or direct drug deposition, and can be localized or widespread. Common drug-induced cutaneous reactions and their clinical presentation will be reviewed in this section.

Often drug-induced skin reactions are difficult to distinguish from common non-drug-related rashes. Therefore, when performing a dermatological assessment, obtaining a medication and allergy history is essential. For patients presenting with a skin rash, review all current and previous prescription medications including OTC medications, herbals, and vaccinations. Identifying the onset of the skin reaction is useful because the onset generally occurs within a few days to weeks from the introduction of the causative agent, for example, starting a new medication. However, medications used for many years can also be the cause. In order to determine the etiology of a drug-related eruption, one must rule out recent exposure to nondrug allergens as the cause of the skin reaction (Law, 2011). Management of skin reactions related to medications primarily involves removing the offending agent; however, corticosteroids, antihistamines, and antipruritic agents may be needed for additional treatment.

Exanthematous (erythematous) drug eruptions are the most common type of adverse skin–drug reaction (**Table 5-10**). It is considered a type IV delayed cell-mediated hypersensitivity reaction. It usually develops 4 to 14 days after initiating a new drug, but the eruption may occur 1 to 2 days after cessation of drug therapy. Presentation of erythematous reactions typically includes **erythema**, also known as skin redness, and maculopapular lesions (**FIGURE 5-24**). These lesions are also known as drug rashes. They often develop on the trunk or upper extremities, and progressively become connected over large areas

Erythema:
Redness of the skin due to congestion of the superficial capillaries.

Table 5-10 Examples of Causes of Exanthematous Drug Reactions

Barbiturates

Carbamazepine

Cephalosporins

Furosemide

Gold salts

Lithium

Penicillin

Phenothiazines

Phenytoin

Sulfonamides

Data from Goeser AL. Skin, hair, and nails. In: Jones RM, Rospond RM, eds. *Patient Assessment in Pharmacy Practice.* 2nd ed. Baltimore, MD: Lippincott Williams & Wilkins; 2009:118–140; Lee A, Thomson J. Drug-induced skin reactions. In: Lee A, ed. *Adverse Drug Reactions.* 2nd ed. London, UK: Pharmaceutical Press; 2006:125–154. Available at: http://www.pharmpress.com/files/docs/ADRe2Ch05.pdf. Accessed March 20, 2013.

of the skin; however, mucous membranes are generally not involved. The rashes may also be associated with pruritus or low-grade fever, which generally resolves in a few days.

Fixed drug eruptions are attributed to drugs or chemicals (**Table 5-11**). These eruptions clinically present as red, raised lesions (**FIGURE 5-25**). These lesions may be pruritic, burn, blister, or turn into plaques. They may occur on any part of the skin, including the mucous membranes. Upon reexposure to the causative agent, the fixed drug eruptions will reoccur in the same location as the previous lesions. These rashes can appear within a few days to weeks after exposure. The lesions disappear a few days after discontinuation of the drug, but leave a residual hyperpigmentation that may take months to fade away.

Urticaria (hives) is a common, acute cutaneous drug reaction. It presents as very pruritic, red, raised wheals that are pale in the center and red around the edges (**FIGURE 5-26**). Edema may also be present. The lesions can vary in number and size, and may be found

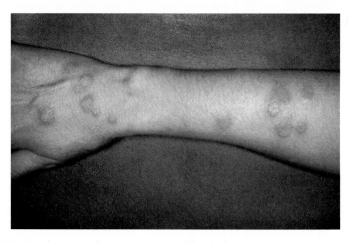

FIGURE 5-24 Exanthematous drug eruption caused by clindamycin.
© Z112/Custom Medical Stock Photo

Table 5-11 Examples of Causes of Fixed Drug Reactions

ACE inhibitors

Allopurinol

Amlodipine

Barbiturates

Benzodiazepine

Carbamazepine

Lamotrigine

Metronidazole

Nonsteroidal anti-inflammatory drugs (NSAIDs)

Penicillin

Sulfonamides

Tetracyclines

Data from Goeser AL. Skin, hair, and nails. In: Jones RM, Rospond RM, eds. *Patient Assessment in Pharmacy Practice.* 2nd ed. Baltimore, MD: Lippincott Williams & Wilkins; 2009:118–140; Lee A, Thomson J. Drug-induced skin reactions. In: Lee A, ed. *Adverse Drug Reactions.* 2nd ed. London, UK: Pharmaceutical Press; 2006:125–154. Available at: http://www.pharmpress.com/files/docs/ADRe2Ch05.pdf. Accessed March 20, 2013.

anywhere on the body. They can appear rapidly within a few hours, but individual lesions rarely persist for more than 24 hours. Angioedema, which may be associated with urticaria, presents as swelling in the subcutaneous or submucosal areas. The tongue, lips, eyelids, extremities, or genitalia are generally affected as well. Both urticaria and angioedema can be complicated by life-threatening anaphylaxis that may involve a variety of organ systems in the body. These urticarial reactions are believed to be caused by an IgE mediated–type hypersensitivity reaction, histamine process, or inflammatory mediators. Management involves discontinuation of the causative agent, sometimes combined with histamine (H_1) receptor blockers. In severe cases of angioedema and anaphylaxis, systemic corticosteroids and epinephrine are given.

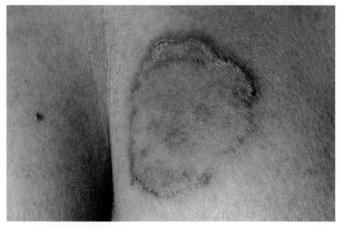

FIGURE 5-25 Fixed drug eruption caused by Bactrim.
© ISM/Phototake, Inc.

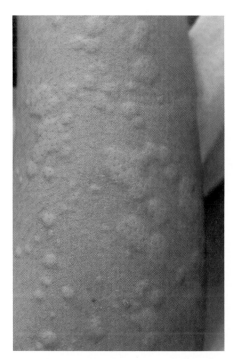

FIGURE 5-26 Urticaria.
© konmesa/iStock/Thinkstock

Stevens-Johnson syndrome (SJS) and toxic epidermal necrolysis (TEN) are rare, severe, life-threatening conditions. Both conditions overlap and may be variants of the same disease. The exact mechanism is unknown but it is believed that SJS and TEN are caused by an immune complex or cell-mediated allergic response. Acute symptoms begin up to 4 weeks (usually 7–21 days) after drug exposure, but can occur a few days after the drug has been withdrawn. Patients typically present with fever and flu-like symptoms

Case #2

MY is a 55-year-old African American man who presents to your clinic with pruritic, erythematous wheals on the trunk of his body. The lesions are 1–2 mm in diameter. He does not have any facial or laryngeal swelling. His symptoms began the previous night. He states yesterday afternoon he started taking amoxicillin for a tooth infection. MY's medical history includes hypertension, diabetes, and depression. His current medications are amlodipine 10 mg daily, metformin 1000 mg BID,

and sertraline 50 mg daily. He has been taking the chronic medications for 3 years.

Questions
1. Is MY's complaint consistent with a drug-induced skin reaction? Which condition?
2. Which of MY's medications is most likely the causative agent?
3. What additional questions would you ask MY to determine if his symptoms are drug related?

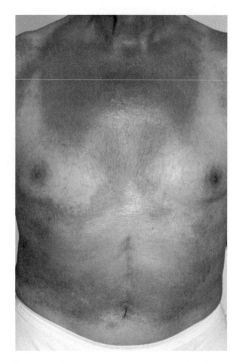

FIGURE 5-27 Photosensitivity reaction causing an exaggerated sunburn appearance.
© John Radcliffe Hospital/Science Source

followed by the development of skin blisters and mucous membrane erosions 1–2 days later. The eruptions appear initially as irregularly shaped, erythematous, purpuric (red-purple in color) macules that progressively merge and lead to skin detachment and sloughing. The lesions begin on the face or upper trunk, but can spread rapidly to cover the entire body. Also, symptoms can manifest internally with sloughing of the intestinal and pulmonary epithelium. SJS is classified as affecting < 10% body surface area (BSA) whereas TEN affects > 30% BSA. HIV-infected patients have a higher risk of developing SJS or TEN. Discontinuation of the offending agent is crucial. Management is symptomatic involving hydration and corticosteroids. Patients experiencing SJS or TEN need to be referred for medical attention immediately.

Drug-induced photosensitivity (**FIGURE 5-27**) reactions can be phototoxic or photo-allergic. They may be caused by topical or systemic medications. Phototoxicity occurs on sun-exposed skin areas causing an exaggerated skin burn, followed by hyperpigmentation. The skin eruption can be localized or widespread, occurring 5–20 hours after sun exposure. Photoallergy is a cell-mediated hypersensitivity reaction, precipitated by ultraviolet radiation, that converts a drug into a photoantigen. Onset can be delayed 24–72 hours, and unlike phototoxicity, it can spread beyond the sun-exposed area. Photoallergy is more of a chronic condition presenting with pruritic, eczematous eruptions. Avoiding direct sunlight, wearing protective clothing, and using sunscreen are recommended to prevent photosensitivity. Topical corticosteroids and systemic antipruritic agents may be useful for management.

Drug-Induced Hair Loss and Growth

Drug therapy can also affect hair growth. Alopecia, discussed earlier, can be caused by a variety of medications. Hair loss can occur during two different phases of the follicle hair cycle. During the growing hair phase, called anagen effluvium, abrupt cessation of hair growth and shedding occurs within days to weeks of drug administration. This is a common adverse effect of chemotherapy. Conversely, in telogen effluvium, or resting hair phase, there is a 2- to 4-month delay in hair loss after initiation of drug treatment. The etiology of hair loss in this stage is more difficult to determine because it can be the result of factors other than medication, such as illness. Hair loss is usually reversible after discontinuation of the offending drug, but it may take several weeks or months for regrowth to occur.

Hirsutism is the excessive growth of coarse hair with masculine characteristics in a female. Androgenic stimulation of hormone-sensitive hair follicles leads to hair growth mostly localized on the lateral areas of the face and back. Drugs commonly responsible for hirsutism are testosterone, anabolic steroids, and oral contraceptives.

Hypertrichosis is also a type of hair growth, but it occurs on areas of the body where hair is short, typically on the face. Changes in hair color and structure have also been noted with chloroquine and chemotherapeutic drug use.

Nail disorders can develop from medication use. A few or all nails can become affected. Nail disorders can be asymptomatic or associated with pain and impaired digital function. Nail abnormalities include horizontal depressions of the nail plate called Beau's lines (**FIGURE 5-28**), brittle nails, onycholysis or separation of the nail from the nail bed, onychomadesis or complete loss of fingernail, and paronychia, which is a red and painful nail fold. Nail changes are usually reversible after drug discontinuation, but recovery may take several months. Nail discoloration and nail bed hyperpigmentation can also occur.

A list of the various drug-induced skin, hair, and nail disorders that can occur is provided in **Table 5-12**.

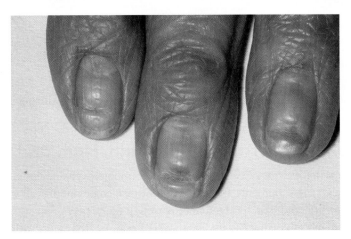

FIGURE 5-28 Beau's lines.
© Dr. P. Marazzi/Science Source

Table 5-12 Types of Drug-Induced Skin, Hair, and Nail Disorders

Disorder	Causes
	Acute Skin Disorders
Erythematous eruptions	Antimicrobials, allopurinol, antiepileptic agents
Urticaria, angioedema, and anaphylaxis	Antimicrobials, NSAIDs, ACE inhibitors, anticancer agents, contrast dye
Fixed-drug eruptions	Antimicrobials, NSAIDs, codeine, barbiturates, calcium channel blockers, proton pump inhibitors
SJS and TEN	Antibacterial sulfonamides, antiepileptic drugs, oxicam and pyrazolone NSAIDs, allopurinol, nevirapine
Photosensitivity	Amiodarone, NSAIDs, thiazides, retinoids, sulfonamides, fluoroquinolones, fibrates, statins, antimalarials, ACE inhibitors
	Chronic Skin Disorders
Drug-induced lupus	*Systemic:* Procainamide, hydralazine isoniazid, methyldopa, minocycline, TNF inhibitors
	Cutaneous: Thiazides, calcium channel blockers, terbinafine, NSAIDs, griseofulvin
Drug-induced acne	Corticosteroids, androgens, lithium, oral contraceptives, isoniazid, azathioprine
Pigmentary changes	*Hyperpigmentation:* Minocycline, antimalarials, amiodarone, oral contraceptives, anticancer drugs
	Hypopigmentation: Topical tretinoin, corticosteroids
	Hair and Nail Disorders
Hair changes	*Hair loss:* Anticancer agents, antidepressants, beta blockers, antithyroid drugs, some antiepileptics, anabolic steroids, lipid-modifying agents, anticoagulants, oral contraceptives
	Hair growth: Minoxidil, testosterone, anabolic steroids, cyclosporine, phenytoin,
Nail changes	Fluoroquinolones, anticancer agents, phenytoin, tetracyclines, thiazides

ACE, angiotensin-converting enzyme; TNF, tumor necrosis factor

Data from Clinard V, Smith JD. Drug-induced skin disorders. *US Pharm.* 2012;37(4):HS11–HS18. Available at: http://www.uspharmacist.com/content/d/feature/c/33698/. Accessed March 20, 2013; Lee A, Thomson J. Drug-induced skin reactions. In: Lee A, ed. *Adverse Drug Reactions.* 2nd ed. London, UK: Pharmaceutical Press; 2006:125–154. Available at: http://www.pharmpress.com/files/docs/ADRe2Ch05.pdf. Accessed March 20, 2013; Valeyrie-Allanore L, Sassolas B, Roujeau JC. Drug-induced skin, nail, and hair disorders. *Drug Saf.* 2007;30: 1011–1030. Available at: http://www.pharmpress.com/files/docs/ADRe2Ch05.pdf. Accessed March 20, 2013.

Cultural Considerations with Skin, Hair, and Nails

Four pigments make up the color of skin: melanin, carotene, oxyhemoglobin, and deoxy-hemoglobin. Of these pigments, melanin is a brownish color and provides the primary coloration for skin and hair. Its abundance is seen in the variety of olives, browns, and tans presented in skin of color (Badueshaia, 2009). Because of the higher melanin content and dispersion, people of color experience lower rates of skin cancer and less pronounced photoaging (Soon, 2009).

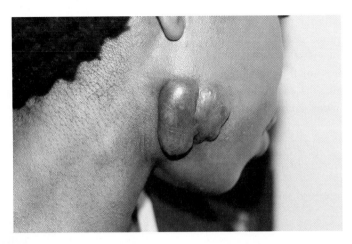

FIGURE 5-29 Keloid.
© Michael Tirgan/Shutterstock, Inc.

Additionally, the presence of increased melanin can lead to differences in clinical presentation of skin conditions. Consequently, skin disorders may be more difficult to diagnose in darker skin tones. Lesions may appear darker, purplish, or grey, instead of red, as typically seen on paler skin. Hyperpigmentation and color demarcations can occur normally on the skin, nail, oral mucosa, and sclera of people of color (Badueshaia, 2009). For example, melanonychia striata or vertical linear streaks on the fingernails is quite common in people of color.

Skin of color contains larger fibroblasts, which can increase the risk for keloids and hypertrophic scars. They often result from wound healing complications from trauma. **Keloids** (**FIGURE 5-29**) may be found anywhere on the body, but generally occur on the ears, chest, neck, upper back, and shoulders. Keloids can present with pruritus, pain, and burning. They initially appear with an erythematous border that turns brownish-red and can pale or darken as they age (Kelly, 2009). Interestingly, in some cultures, fraternal organizations take special care to "brand" their members by forming keloids on various parts of the body. The keloids are purposely placed and specially formed into symbols representing the organizations. Treatment of keloids can be with steroid injections or surgical removal. Hypertrophic scars (**FIGURE 5-30**) appear similar to keloids, but are asymptomatic and may fade over time (Kelly, 2009). Hair is absent from these skin growths.

A particular hyperpigmentation commonly seen in people of color who also have a tendency toward diabetes is known as **acanthosis nigricans** (**FIGURE 5-31**). Generally located on the neck or axillae, these dark brown to black plaques are seen in the folds of skin. It is strongly associated with obesity and insulin resistance (Kelly, 2009). Only recently defined, maturational hyperpigmentation is also associated with obesity and insulin resistance; however, this hyperpigmentation occurs unilaterally or bilaterally on the face. It, too, exhibits as a dark brown to black presentation, but eventually fades into the patient's typical skin color. Often over-the-counter skin creams and bleaches are ineffective, but resolution of the offending hyperpigmentation can be seen with weight loss.

Dermatosis papulosa nigra (**FIGURE 5-32**), also known as skin tags, is an extremely common occurrence on the skin of persons of color (Glen, 2009). Its prevalence is reported

Keloids:
Elevated, irregular scar of fibrous tissue formed at a site of injury.

Acanthosis nigricans:
Brown to black, irregular, velvety hyperpigmentation of the skin often found in folds of the body.

to be high. Although this condition is generally asymptomatic, it can adversely affect cosmetic appearance with its numerous papules. Frequently occurring on the face, neck, and trunk, the growths can be smooth and round, as well as projectile and filliform. As the patient ages and the subsequent papules multiply, they can present with tens to hundreds of papules that can eventually coalesce into larger plaques. The papules and plaques are generally not removed unless they become tender, pruritic, or irritated, generally

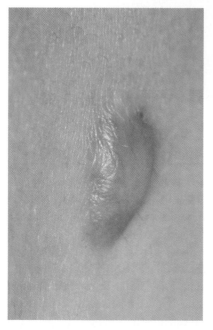

FIGURE 5-30 Hypertrophic scar.
© schankz/Shutterstock, Inc.

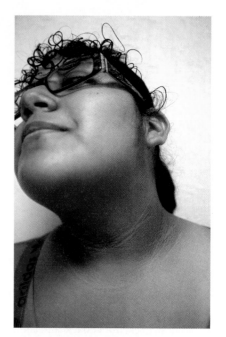

FIGURE 5-31 Acanthosis nigricans.
© Benedicte Desrus/Alamy

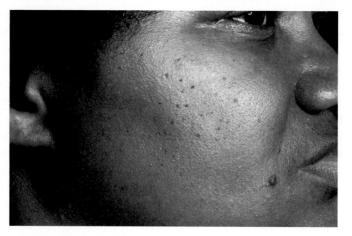

FIGURE 5-32 Dermatosis papulosa nigra.
© Wellcome Image Library/Custom Medical Stock Photo

by clothing. Patients with particularly numerous and sudden papules should be further triaged to exclude any dermatologic malignancies. Relatively simple office treatment is available for patients who desire it; however, care should be taken to avoid scarring, hyper/hypopigmentation, or permanent damage from removal.

Melanomas in persons of color are significantly less common; however, they are usually more advanced when diagnosed and have a poorer prognosis (Soon, 2009). Caucasians present with melanomas on the head and neck, and to a lesser extent on the trunk and legs, whereas their darker-skinned counterparts often present with melanomas on palms, soles, and nail beds. Moreover, because basal cell carcinomas can be pigmented in people of color, they can often be mistaken for seborrheic keratosis. Therefore, a thorough skin examination should be conducted in darker-skinned people suspected of basal cell carcinoma.

Finally, although scientists have found no biochemical differences in the hair of various ethnicities, it has been identified that the manner of care can be associated with alopecia and other pathologies (Quinn, 2009). In particular, black hair can vary from tightly coiled to very straight; however, it has been determined that hair with a tighter curl is more susceptible to breakage. These patients can present with alopecia secondary to straightening, combing, chemical relaxers, braids, weaving, and other cosmetic treatments. Traction alopecia (**FIGURE 5-33**) is rather common in African American girls and women who wear tightly coiffed styles. In general, African Americans shampoo only once or twice weekly, because shampooing more often can lead to dryness and breakage. Many patients utilize pomades, scalp oils, and moisturizers, because the hair does not collect sebum as more naturally straight hair does. These products can ease in detangling and styling. Unfortunately, these products also can lead to an increased prevalence of comedones on the face and neck. Extra precaution should be taken to avoid thermal burns from irons often used to straighten and curl hair. Covered rubber bands without metal hinges can be used to minimize breakage. Chemical relaxers should not be left on too long, to prevent scalp burns. Weaves and braids should be loosened so as not to pull too tightly on the scalp. With proper care and the lack of permanent damage, hair should be able to grow back over time.

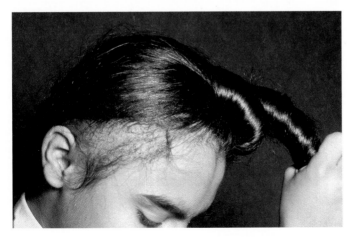

FIGURE 5-33 Traction alopecia.
© Wellcome Image Library/Custom Medical Stock Photo

Pseudofolliculitis barbae:
Razor bumps; persistent irritation caused by shaving.

Men of color with tight, curly facial hair also can experience a common condition called **pseudofolliculitis barbae** (**FIGURE 5-34**). When the area is shaved, the sharpened hairs can curl back into the skin causing inflammation (Kelly, 2009). The papules with hair in the center can become infected. If left untreated and chronic, it can result in permanently scarred areas. This can also occur on the legs and groin if they, too, are shaved closely. Although this condition can occur in any person, people of color are more susceptible due to the nature of the coarser, curlier hair's ability to penetrate the skin. Several preventative measures can be taken such as using electric clippers, using an emollient shaving cream, searching for ingrown hairs prior to shaving, brushing the beard in one direction, using sharp razors and soothing aftershaves, and the like. Similarly, a dermatologic condition called acne keloidalis (**FIGURE 5-35**) can occur in dark-skinned men who shave the posterior neck region (Kelly, 2009). Initially beginning as an acute folliculitis after shaving, it progresses to chronic papules and can result in keloid lesions that grow no hair at the nape of the neck. Those who have this condition should avoid clippers or razors in the

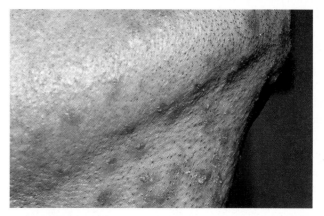

FIGURE 5-34 Pseudofolliculitis barbae.
© Dr. Allan Harris/Phototake

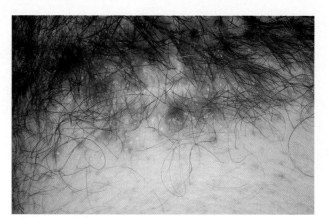

FIGURE 5-35 Acne keloidalis.
© Dr. Hercules Robinson/Phototake

Case #3

JF is a 41-year-old African American man with a diagnosis of new onset type 2 diabetes. He comes to your pharmacy to get his new medications filled, but also inquires about remedies for the darkened areas along the side of his face and around his neck under his shirt collar. He does not like the darkened areas and reports using several facial cleansers with limited results. He also reports that he has used skin bleachers containing hydroquinone, but reports no resolution.

Questions
1. Based on JF's clinical presentation, what condition is most likely present?
2. What disease state(s) are associated with this condition?
3. How should patients be monitored for resolution?

region and hats or shirts that can further irritate the area. Multiple medical modalities are available for treatment.

Summary

The pharmacist often serves as the patient's first point of contact and initial screener with a healthcare professional due to their ease of accessibility in the community setting. The visibility of the skin, hair, and nails allows for a quick and easy assessment of cutaneous conditions. Many dermatological disorders, including some drug-induced reactions, can be appropriately managed with a pharmacist's recommendation. Additionally, persons of color can exhibit varied presentations of the same disorder secondary to skin coloration. Because of the darkened skin, clinical presentation may be different and pathologies may be less noticeable; therefore, closer inspection is warranted to view the affected area. Special consideration must also be given to hair and skin care in people of color. Some products and treatments can cause irritation, swelling, hair loss, and permanent scarring.

Review Questions

1. Compare and contrast exanthematous drug reactions, fixed drug reactions, and urticaria.
2. Explain how the clinical presentation of contact dermatitis differs from the clinical presentation of fungal skin infections.
3. How do melanomas present differently in persons of color?
4. Differentiate potential differences in hair care for people of color. How can these differences potentially manifest in pathologies?

References

Alexander AM. Maturational hyperpigmentation. In: Kelly AP, Taylor SC, eds. *Dermatology for Skin of Color*. New York: McGraw-Hill; 2009:344.

American Academy of Dermatology. Melanoma: Signs and symptoms. Available at: http://www.aad.org/dermatology-a-to-z/diseases-and-treatments/m—p/melanoma/signs-symptoms. Accessed March 21, 2013.

Badreshia-Bansal S, Taylor SC. The structure and function of skin of color. In: Kelly AP, Taylor SC, eds. *Dermatology for Skin of Color*. New York: McGraw-Hill; 2009:71–77.

Bernard DB. Minor burns, sunburn, and wounds. In: Berardi RR, Ferreri SP, Hume AL, et al., eds. *Handbook of Nonprescription Drugs: An Interactive Approach to Self-Care*. 17th ed. Washington, DC: American Pharmacists Association; 2009:735–755.

Berry TM. Hair loss. In: Berardi RR, Ferreri SP, Hume AL, et al., eds. *Handbook of Nonprescription Drugs: An Interactive Approach to Self-Care*. 17th ed. Washington, DC: American Pharmacists Association; 2009:811–821.

Bickley LS, Szilagyi P. The skin, hair, and nails. In: Bickley LS, Szilagyi P, eds. *Bates' Guide to Physical Examination and History Taking*. 10th ed. Philadelphia, PA: Lippincott Williams & Wilkins; 2009:163–190.

Clinard V, Smith JD. Drug-induced skin disorders. *US Pharm*. 2012;37(4):HS11–HS18. Available at: http://www.uspharmacist.com/content/d/feature/c/33698/. Accessed March 20, 2013.

DeSimone EM. Skin, hair, and nails. In: Jones RM, Rospond RM, eds. *Patient Assessment in Pharmacy Practice*. 1st ed. Baltimore, MD: Lippincott Williams & Wilkins; 2002:102–128.

Forman SB, Garrett, AB. Basal cell carcinoma. In: Kelly AP, Taylor SC, eds. *Dermatology for Skin of Color*. New York: McGraw-Hill; 2009:296–299.

Glen MJ. Dermatosis papulosa nigra. In: Kelly AP, Taylor SC, eds. *Dermatology for Skin of Color*. New York: McGraw-Hill; 2009:552–554.

Goeser AL. Skin, hair, and nails. In: Jones RM, Rospond RM, eds. *Patient Assessment in Pharmacy Practice*. 2nd ed. Baltimore, MD: Lippincott Williams & Wilkins; 2009: 118–140.

Kelly AP. Acne keloidalis. In: Kelly AP, Taylor SC, eds. *Dermatology for Skin of Color*. New York: McGraw-Hill; 2009:205–210.

Kelly AP. Keloids. In: Kelly AP, Taylor SC, eds. *Dermatology for Skin of Color*. New York: McGraw-Hill; 2009:178–194.

Kelly AP. Pseudofolliculitis barbae. In: Kelly AP, Taylor SC, eds. *Dermatology for Skin of Color*. New York: McGraw-Hill; 2009:211–216.

Law RM, Law DT. Dermatologic drug reactions and common skin conditions. In: Talbert RL, DiPiro JT, Matzke GR, Posey LM, Wells BG, Yee GC, eds. *Pharmacotherapy: A Pathophysiologic Approach*. 8th ed. New York: McGraw-Hill; 2011. Available at: http://www.accesspharmacy.com/content.aspx?aID=7998475. Accessed April 6, 2013.

Lee A, Thomson J. Drug-induced skin reactions. In: Lee A, ed. *Adverse Drug Reactions*. 2nd ed. London, UK: Pharmaceutical Press; 2006:125–154. Available at: http://www.pharmpress .com/files/docs/ADRe2Ch05.pdf. Accessed March 20, 2013.

Lehmann HP, Robinson KA, Andrews JS, Holloway V, Goodman SN. Acne therapy: A methodologic review. *J Am Acad Dermatol*. 2002;47:231–240.

McKinley-Grant L, Warnick M, Singh, S. Cutaneous manifestations of systemic diseases. In: Kelly AP, Taylor SC, eds. *Dermatology for Skin of Color*. New York: McGraw-Hill; 2009:178–194.

National Cancer Institute. Common moles, dysplastic nevi, and risk of melanoma. Available at: http://www.cancer.gov/cancertopics/factsheet/Risk/moles. Accessed April 5, 2013.

Newton G, Zweber A. OTC advisor: Self-care dermatologic disorders. American Pharmacists Association. Available at: http://elearning.pharmacist.com/Portal/Files/Learning Products/514b8af7d93d4cfdae01eb41f2b73b36/assets/037_OTC%20Advisor_Derm _FINAL.pdf. Accessed May 17, 2014.

Newton GD, Popovich NG. Fungal skin infections. In: Berardi RR, Ferreri SP, Hume AL, et al., eds. *Handbook of Nonprescription Drugs: An Interactive Approach to Self-Care.* 17th ed. Washington, DC: American Pharmacists Association; 2009:775–789.

Plake KS, Darbishire PL. Contact dermatitis. In: Berardi RR, Ferreri SP, Hume AL, et al., eds. *Handbook of Nonprescription Drugs: An Interactive Approach to Self-Care.* 17th ed. Washington, DC: American Pharmacists Association; 2009:657–673.

Quairoli K, Foster KT. Acne. In: Berardi RR, Ferreri SP, Hume AL, et al., eds. *Handbook of Nonprescription Drugs: An Interactive Approach to Self-Care.* 17th ed. Washington, DC: American Pharmacists Association; 2009:707–717.

Quinn CR. Hair care practices. In: Kelly AP, Taylor SC, eds. *Dermatology for Skin of Color.* New York: McGraw-Hill; 2009:217–226.

Scott SA. Atopic dermatitis and dry skin. In: Berardi RR, Ferreri SP, Hume AL, et al., eds. *Handbook of Nonprescription Drugs: An Interactive Approach to Self-Care.* 17th ed. Washington, DC: American Pharmacists Association; 2009:627–642.

Seidel HM, Ball JW, Dains JE, Benedict GW, eds. *Mosby's Guide to Physical Examination.* 6th ed. St. Louis, MO: Elsevier; 2006:169–229.

Sibbald D. Acne vulgaris. In: Talbert RL, DiPiro JT, Matzke GR, Posey LM, Wells BG, Yee GC, eds. *Pharmacotherapy: A Pathophysiologic Approach.* 8th ed. New York: McGraw-Hill; 2011. Available at: http://www.accesspharmacy.com/content.aspx?aID =7998615. Accessed April 6, 2013.

Singer AJ. Thermal burns: Rapid assessment and treatment. *Emerg Med Pract.* 2000;2(9):1–20. Available at: http://www.ebmedicine.net/topics.php?paction=showTopicSeg&topic _id=111&seg_id=2135. Accessed March 2, 2014.

Soon SL, Washington CV. Melanoma in skin of color. In: Kelly AP, Taylor SC, eds. *Dermatology for Skin of Color.* New York: McGraw-Hill; 2009:283–290.

Valeyrie-Allanore L, Sassolas B, Roujeau JC. Drug-induced skin, nail, and hair disorders. *Drug Saf.* 2007;30:1011–1030. Available at: http://www.pharmpress.com/files/docs/ ADRe2Ch05.pdf. Accessed March 20, 2013.

Chapter 6

Head and Neck Assessment
Yolanda M. Hardy, PharmD

LEARNING OBJECTIVES

At the completion of this chapter, the reader should be able to:

1. Explain the clinical presentation of common disease processes related to the head and neck.
2. Determine the appropriate questions to ask patients when performing a focused interview related to the head and neck.
3. Explain observation techniques utilized in assessing head and neck conditions.
4. Triage patients based on clinical presentation of problems related to the head and neck.
5. List medications that can cause adverse drug events and medical processes related to the head and neck.
6. Explain the clinical presentation of drug-induced medical processes.
7. Describe cultural concepts related to causes and management of headache.

KEY TERMS

Allergic crease	Allergic shiners	Secondary headache
Allergic face	Moon facies	
Allergic salute	Primary headache	

Introduction

This chapter will discuss conditions related to the head and neck that the pharmacist may encounter while working with clients. Many of the conditions related to the head and neck that a pharmacist will encounter can be assessed by patient interview and not physical assessment. Thus, most of this chapter will focus on questions to ask the patient. The patient interview for all of the conditions presented should include questions that will allow you to gather information regarding the following areas: onset, location, duration, character, aggravating factors, relieving factors, timing,

© ontishock/Shutterstock, Inc.

and severity. However, in some instances, being able to recognize certain signs by observation will be important in determining the appropriate next steps in care for the patient. Situations where the ability to observe certain signs is important will be highlighted as well.

Clinical Presentation of Disease Processes of the Head and Neck

Headache

Headache is a common symptom that pharmacists encounter in the outpatient setting. A headache can be a symptom of a minor problem such as not getting enough rest or a major problem such as an aneurysm (Bickley & Szilagyi, 2009; Kaniecki, 2003; Goadsby & Raskin, 2012). A thorough history is necessary to help with determining whether the headache can be managed by the patient or if further management by a physician is needed.

Headaches can be classified as a primary headache or a secondary headache. Headaches due to an unknown cause are considered **primary headaches**. Migraine headaches, tension-type headaches, and cluster headaches are common primary headaches (Bickley & Szilagyi, 2009; Kaniecki, 2003; Goadsby & Raskin, 2012; Wood, 2011). Each of these types of headaches has a different clinical presentation and somewhat different treatment options (**FIGURE 6-1**). Headaches due to an underlying cause are called **secondary headaches** (Bickley & Szilagyi, 2009; Kaniecki, 2003; Goadsby & Raskin, 2012; Wood, 2011). Secondary headaches warrant treatment by a healthcare provider and should not be managed by the patient unless under the supervision of the provider.

Primary headache: A headache in which the underlying cause is unknown.

Secondary headache: A headache in which the underlying cause is known.

The Patient Interview

The pharmacist can differentiate among the three types of headaches as well as determine if self-care treatment is warranted solely by performing a patient interview using the core questions. Quality information regarding the patient's concern can be discerned without performing a physical assessment. As the pharmacist is listening to the patient's responses, he or she should be aware of responses that would suggest follow-up care with a primary care provider or immediate emergency care (**FIGURE 6-2**). If the patient responds with such answers about the headache, the pharmacist can ask further questions to help determine the most appropriate referral. For example, if a patient reports experiencing a head injury in the immediate past for which treatment was not sought, and is now complaining of additional symptoms such as dizziness and blurred vision, it may be more appropriate to refer that patient for emergency treatment (Pray, 2009; Remington, 2006).

Conjunctivitis

Conjunctivitis is simply defined as inflammation of the conjunctiva of the eye. Causes of conjunctivitis may be infectious in nature or due to allergy or irritation (Horton, 2012). Conjunctivitis can affect neonates, infants, children, and adults. The most common characteristics of conjunctivitis are a red eye and discharge or drainage from the eye; however, other signs and symptoms differ based on the cause of the inflamed conjunctiva (Hortin, 2012; Leibowitz, 2000) (**FIGURE 6-3**).

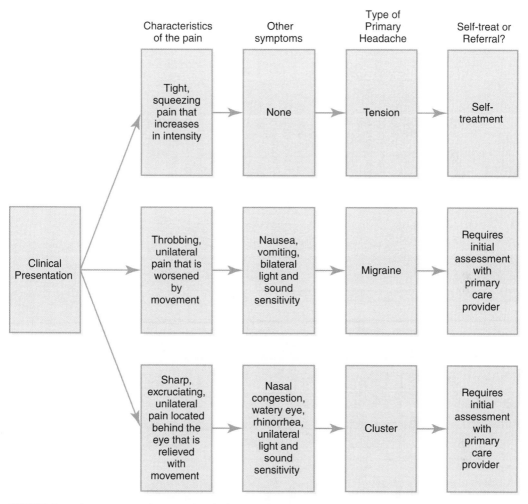

FIGURE 6-1 Characteristics of primary headaches.

Data from Remington T. Headache. In: Berardi R, Ferreri S, Hume A, Kroon L, Newton, G, Popovich N., et al., eds. *Handbook of Nonprescription Drugs: An Interactive Approach to Self-Care.* 16th ed. Washington, DC: American Pharmacists Association; 2009;69–90 and Scott C. An introduction to diagnosis and management of headache. *Nurs Stand.* 2011;26:35–38.

Responses That Warrant Follow-up or Immediate Care
1) Recent reports of head injury or trauma
2) First time experiencing a headache
3) Complaints of "the worst headache in my life"
4) Symptoms of dizziness, vision loss, or vomiting
5) Symptoms worsen rather than get better
6) Onset of headaches begin after the age of 50
7) Headache precipitated by exertion or exercise
8) Sudden onset described as a "clap"
9) Headache during pregnancy or postpartum
10) Headache that awakens the person from sleeping

FIGURE 6-2 Responses that warrant follow up with a primary care provider or immediate care.

Data from Pray W. Patients with headaches: The pharmacist's role. *US Pharm.* 2009;34:12–15.

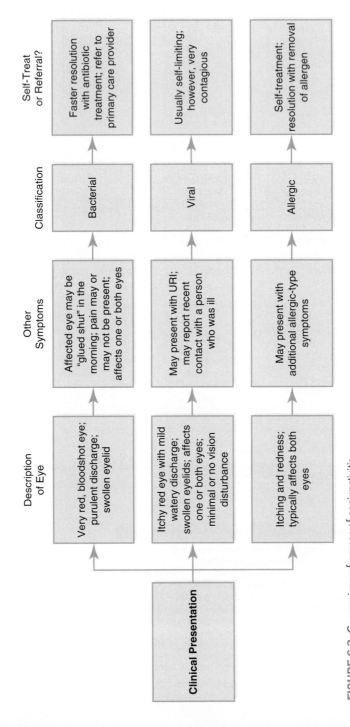

FIGURE 6-3 Comparison of causes of conjunctivitis.

Data from Leibowitz H. The red eye. *New Engl J Med.* 2000;343(5):345–351.

Responses That Warrant Medical Treatment
1) Blurry vision
2) Chemical or heat exposure to the eye
3) Loss of vision
4) Pain
5) Reports of recent injury to the eye
6) Symptoms lasting more than 3 days

FIGURE 6-4 Responses that warrant medical treatment.

Data from Fiscella R, Jensen M. Ophthalmic disorders. In: Berardi R, Kroon LA, McDermott JH, Newton GD, Oszko MA, Popovich N., et al., eds. *Handbook of Nonprescription Drugs: An Interactive Approach to Self-Care.* 15th ed. Washington, DC: American Pharmacists Association; 2006:577–604.

Although patients may refer to a red eye as "pink eye," this term is usually used to describe infectious conjunctivitis caused by a virus (Albrecht, 2011; Fiscella, 2009; Horton, 2012; Leibowitz, 2000; Tarabishy, 2008).

The Patient Interview

When a patient presents to the pharmacist with complaints of a red, irritated eye, the pharmacist can perform a patient interview to help determine if the patient can self-manage the condition or if the patient should seek medical treatment (**FIGURE 6-4**). In addition to the core questions mentioned in the introduction to this chapter, the pharmacist should ask about discharge from the eye and the quality of the discharge. Because discharge that results in the eye being glued shut in the morning has been found to be highly indicative of bacterial conjunctivitis, the pharmacist should be sure to ask about this particular characteristic. In addition, the pharmacist should inquire about recent injury to the eye (Rietveld, 2004). Last, the pharmacist should ask about contact lens use and hygiene, as well as use of eye makeup, because improperly cleaned contacts or eye makeup and instruments used to apply the makeup may harbor bacteria, which could lead to infection. Asking about recent changes in contact brands or solutions and about use of new eye makeup, facial creams, or lotions is important because symptoms developing after use of a new product may suggest an allergic response (Fiscella, 2009).

Physical Exam Findings

A pharmacist will rarely perform an eye exam on a patient; however, it is important for a pharmacist to be able to look at a person's eye to determine if there is a problem. Key findings from observing a patient's eye would include redness of the conjunctiva and the inside area of the eyelid (**FIGURE 6-5**).

Case #1

SJ presents to the pharmacy counter wishing to purchase allergy eye drops for her eyes. As you are speaking with SJ, you notice that her left eye is red and somewhat swollen, and that she uses a tissue to clean off a liquid discharge from her eye. Her right eye does not appear to be affected.

Questions

1. What questions should you ask SJ regarding her eye condition?
2. What question would you ask to determine if this is possibly bacterial conjunctivitis?

A.

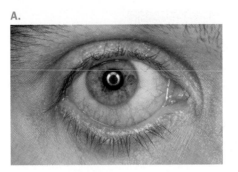

B.

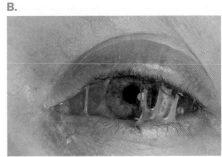

FIGURE 6-5 A. Conjunctivitis. B. Bacterial conjunctivitis.

A. © Pavel L Photo and Video/ShutterStock. B. © TimMcCleqn/iStockphoto

Otitis Media

Otitis media, also referred to as an ear infection, commonly is seen in the pediatric population, though adults can be affected as well. Otitis media can be classified as either acute otitis media or otitis media with effusion. Otitis media can occur after a viral upper respiratory tract infection (Rubin, 2012; Shaikh & Hoberman, 2010); however, even in these cases, the cause of the ear infection is a bacterial infection. Otitis media with effusion is characterized by the presence of fluid in the Eustachian tube that has not properly drained from the tube (Rubin, 2012; Shaikh & Hoberman, 2010). Signs and symptoms of otitis media can include fever, headache, irritability, runny nose, cough, decreased appetite, and diarrhea. Otalgia, or ear pain, is another symptom that may be present.

The Patient Interview

In the majority of cases, the pharmacist will be discussing this problem with the parent of the child presenting with the aforementioned symptoms. The presenting symptoms of an ear infection are similar to those of other medical conditions, such as an upper respiratory tract infection; as a result, an additional question to ask the parent is about the presence of ear pain. Children who may be too young to express pain may be seen pulling or rubbing at the affected ear (Ramakrishnan, 2007). Asking a parent if he or she has noticed this type of behavior in the child will be helpful in determining if the symptoms are related to an ear infection.

Physical Exam Findings

Ear infections are diagnosed in part by the characteristics of the symptoms, but also by inspection of the tympanic membrane. The role of the pharmacist in the assessment of otitis media would most likely *not* include inspecting the ear for the presence of inflammation or effusion; rather, it would be to refer the patient and parent to seek further analysis by the primary care provider when otitis media is suspected.

Treatment methods for otitis media include delaying the initiation of antibiotics in order to see if the infection will resolve on its own (Ramakrishnan, 2007; Rubin, 2012). Although this method is used, it should not be initiated by the pharmacist unless the pharmacist is working in a specialized area related to ear conditions and perhaps under the guidance of a collaborative practice agreement. In other instances, this method is not used and antibiotics are initiated upon clinical presentation of symptoms.

Rhinosinusitis

Rhinosinusitis is characterized by inflammation of the sinus cavities and the nasal mucosa. It can be of an infectious (viral, bacterial, or fungal) or noninfectious origin. Noninfectious and viral forms of rhinosinusitis are self-limiting, and can be treated using self-care practices. Bacterial rhinosinusitis and chronic sinusitis should be evaluated by a healthcare provider. Rhinosinusitis can be classified as acute, subacute, or chronic. These classifications are based on the length of time the patient is experiencing the condition (Georgy, 2012; Rubin, 2012).

Common symptoms of rhinosinusitis include nasal congestion, purulent or bloody nasal discharge, nasal stuffiness, facial pressure, and headache. Some patients may also report tooth pain and decreased sense of smell. Cough, fatigue, fever, and bad breath can also be symptoms of this condition (Georgy, 2012; Rubin, 2012).

The Patient Interview

When assessing rhinosinusitis, the pharmacist should ask the patient questions related to recent illnesses, in particular recent upper respiratory tract infections. Asking about the duration of symptoms is important because symptoms presenting for longer than 7–10 days suggest a bacterial infection, for which the patient should be referred to the primary care provider for further assessment and possibly antibiotic therapy (Rubin, 2012; Georgy, 2012). Symptoms lasting for more than 12 weeks suggest chronic sinusitis, which also should be evaluated by the patient's primary care physician.

Physical Exam Findings

There are a few unique techniques that a pharmacist can have the patient perform when they present with symptoms suggestive of sinusitis. Facial pressure related to sinusitis can often worsen when the patient bends over or makes a postural change in position (Scolaro, 2009). Asking the patient to bend over as if picking something up from the floor and reporting the presence of facial pain is an assessment the pharmacist can perform.

Case #2

CR is a 40-year-old man who presents to the pharmacy to pick up medication for his son. While there, he mentions to you that he has been experiencing a stuffy nose and a dull headache for the past 2 weeks. He states that he has been taking pain relievers for the headache, but it doesn't go away. You suspect that he may have rhinosinusitis.

Question
1. What additional questions would you ask CR to determine if he is experiencing rhinosinusitis?

Case #2 *(continued)*

CR tells you that he has noticed some streaks of blood when he blows his nose. He states that he seems to have lost his sense of smell, and though he has not noticed any tooth pain, his wife told him that his breath smells different, almost unpleasant. You ask CR to bend down as if he were picking up something from the floor and report any pain. He tells you that he notices pain on his forehead.

Questions

2. Is CR's complaint consistent with rhinosinusitis? Why?
3. What would be your recommendation for CR? Why?

Allergic Rhinitis

Allergic rhinitis is the inflammation of the nasal mucosa. Patients commonly call this condition "hay fever" or "allergies." Symptoms related to allergic rhinitis include itching of the nose, sneezing, nasal congestion, and rhinorrhea. Allergic rhinitis can be classified as intermittent, occurring less than 4 days a week or less than 4 consecutive weeks, or persistent, in which the patient experiences symptoms more than 4 days a week and for more than 4 weeks consistently (Brozek, 2010; Uzzman, 2012).

The Patient Interview

Asking the core questions related to onset, location, duration, character, aggravating factors, relieving factors, timing, and severity can help the pharmacist discern if the patient is suffering from intermittent or persistent allergic rhinitis, as well as help identify the causative allergen.

The Physical Exam

The physical exam technique that the pharmacist can employ is primarily observation of the patient. In addition to the common symptoms of allergic rhinitis, patients may also display various other signs of this condition. **Allergic shiners** (**FIGURE 6-6A**), which are described as dark circles under the eyes—as if the person has a black eye—is a common symptom seen in children and teenagers with allergic rhinitis. The **allergic salute** (**FIGURE 6-6B**) is also a sign that can be seen. This is the act of rubbing the nose in an upward manner using the open palm of the hand. The **allergic face** (**FIGURE 6-6C**) is described as a face with a droopy, tired, and even swollen appearance. This is due to swelling of the adenoids in the back of the throat. The **allergic crease** (**FIGURE 6-6D**) is described as a series of lines that run horizontally across the bridge of the nose (American College of Allergy, Asthma, and Immunology). This is commonly seen in children, and is a result of multiple allergic salutes. Mouth breathing is also a common sign, as a result of the nasal congestion experienced by the patient.

Because allergic rhinitis is quite common, patients will often initiate treatment of this condition without seeking the help of a healthcare provider. However, if a patient reports symptoms that fail to respond to over-the-counter treatments or complains of symptoms after identification and removal of offending allergens, then a referral to the primary care provider may be warranted.

Mouth Sores

Two common conditions that affect the mouth, and are sometimes confused with each other, are aphthous ulcers, also referred to as canker sores, and cold sores or *Herpes labialis*, also referred to as fever blisters. Canker sores are painful sores that can present in the mucosal area of the mouth. These sores are round and white or yellow. A patient

---

Allergic shiners:
Dark circles presenting beneath the eye cavities.

Allergic salute:
The action in which the tip of the nose is rubbed in an upward motion, usually with the palm of the hand.

Allergic face:
Facial presentation characterized by facial swelling, darkness around the eyes, and open-mouthed breathing. Patient may also appear fatigued.

Allergic crease:
A horizontal line seen across the bridge of the nose that results from repetitively rubbing the tip of the nose in an upward fashion.

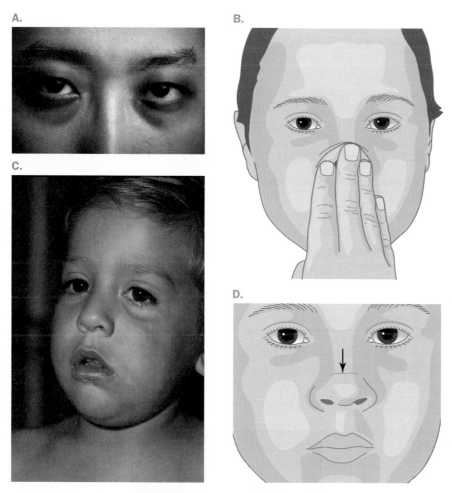

FIGURE 6-6 A. Allergic shiner. B. Allergic salute. C. Allergic face. D. Allergic crease.

A. © szefei/ShutterStock. C. © Schleickorn/Custom Medical Stock Photo

can present with one ulcer or multiple ulcers at a time. Because of the pain associated with canker sores, they can cause problems with eating or speaking. These sores are not associated with fever, gastrointestinal symptoms, or the presence of similar looking sores on the skin.

Cold sores, on the other hand, are painful sores caused by the herpes simplex virus (Gonsalves, 2007; McBride, 2000; Messadi, 2010). They appear on the outside of the mouth, either on the lips or close to the lip area. Cold sores initially present with a prodromal stage, in which the patient will experience an itching or tingling sensation beginning a few days before the vesicular cluster of sores appears. Within 1–2 days of appearing, the vesicles will rupture, form an ulcer, and then crust over (Gonsalves, 2007).

The Patient Interview

Questions related to mouth sores should focus on the core questions mentioned earlier. In addition, asking about the presence of other symptoms is important, because the presence of other symptoms may suggest another condition and may warrant referral to the primary care provider or dentist. Because cold sores can be precipitated by stress, illness, temperature changes, excess sun exposure, or a weakened immune system, asking about these things is important in the patient interview (Usatine, 2010). Both conditions, in their mild forms, are self-limiting and do not warrant a visit to the primary care provider. However, patients that are immunocompromised or present with other symptoms such as gastrointestinal symptoms, other sores on the skin, or other symptoms that are not related to these conditions should be referred for further workup (Gonsalves, 2007; McBride, 2000; Messadi, 2010).

Clinical Presentation of Drug-Induced Processes

Often, a patient will present with signs and symptoms suggestive of a disease; however, after evaluation, it is discovered that the clinical presentation is actually the result of medication use. Pharmacists can be a tremendous help to the medical team when we consider the possibility of drug-related causes for a patient's condition. As a result, being aware of and assessing patients for drug-related causes of the clinical presentation is a very valuable skill.

Moon Facies

Moon facies:
A condition in which the face takes on a full round shape. Can be seen in Cushing's syndrome or as a result of long-term use of high dose corticosteroids.

Moon facies is a sign seen in Cushing's syndrome, a condition caused by exposure to high levels of corticosteroids. This high exposure can be due to excess secretion of adreno-corticotropic hormone (ACTH) from the pituitary gland or chronic use of high doses of systemic corticosteroids (Else, 2010). Cushing's syndrome due to systemic steroids is called iatrogenic Cushing's syndrome. A person with moon facies will have a rounder face resembling the round shape of the moon. This change in shape of the head is due to fat redistribution as a result of the exposure to high levels of corticosteroids (**FIGURE 6-7**).

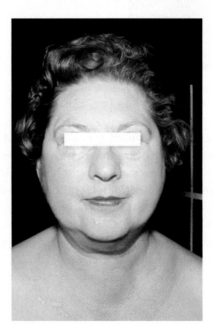

FIGURE 6-7 Moon facies.
Courtesy of Leonard V. Crowley, MD, Century College.

Nystagmus

Nystagmus is characterized as a repetitive movement of the eyes. Medications associated with causing nystagmus include carbamazepine, dextromethorphan, ethanol, ketamine, lithium, monoamine oxidase inhibitors, phencyclidine, phenytoin, and sedative hypnotics (Sharma, 2011). This sign can be indicative of toxicity due to high doses of these medications. An assessment for nystagmus can be performed rather quickly (Bickley, 2009; Rospond, 2003) (Table 6-1).

Table 6-1 Assessment for Nystagmus

Stand in front of the patient.

Ask the patient to follow the movement of your finger using only his or her eyes. The patient's head should continue to stay in the forward position.

Place your finger about 12 inches or a little further from the patient's face. Begin to move your finger to the patient's right.

While on the patient's right side, proceed to move the finger upward, and then downward on the right side.

Move your finger back toward the front center of the patient's face, and then continue to move to the left side.

Repeat the same process on the left side.

Observe the patient's eyes during the process for involuntary or jerking movements.

Data from Jones R, Rospond R. *Patient Assessment in Pharmacy Practice*. Philadelphia, PA: Lippincott, Williams & Wilkins; 2003: 129–156.

Tinnitus

Tinnitus is the perception of sound although sound is not present. It may be described by patients as a ringing in the ear. Tinnitus may or may not be associated with hearing loss. In general, the incidence of drug-induced tinnitus is low; however, tinnitus has been associated with a number of different medications (Chiang, 2011) (Table 6-2).

Table 6-2 Medications Associated with Tinnitus

Over-the-Counter Agents	Prescription Agents
Antihistamines	Anticonvulsants (carbamazepine, valproic acid) Cardiac (quinidine, lidocaine)
Nonsteroidal anti-inflammatory drugs (NSAIDs)	Antidepressants (amitriptyline, lithium) Diuretics (bumetanide, ethacrynic acid, furosemide, torsemide)
Salicylates (e.g., aspirin)	Anti-infectives (amphotericin B, aminoglycosides, chloroquine, clindamycin, hydroxychloroquine, metronidazole, tetracyclines, vancomycin) Local anesthetics (bupivacaine, lidocaine)
	Antineoplastics (cisplatin, methotrexate, vinblastine, vincristine)

Data from Chiang WK. Chapter 20. Otolaryngologic principles. In: Chiang WK, ed. *Goldfrank's Toxicologic Emergencies*. 9th ed. New York: McGraw-Hill; 2011. http://www.accesspharmacy.com/content.aspx?aID=6506418. Accessed February 23, 2013.

Rhinitis Medicamentosa

Rhinitis medicamentosa is caused by prolonged use of topical nasal decongestants (Graf, 2005; Kushnir, 2013; Ramey et al., 2006). Often, patients who have the problem have been using topical nasal decongestants as a way to treat allergic rhinitis. This condition is characterized by nasal stuffiness and congestion. Patients with this condition will believe that the increased symptoms are related to allergic rhinitis, and as a result will use more of the topical nasal decongestant, hence worsening the problem. Assessing a patient for this condition should include asking the patient if he or she has noticed that the symptoms of nasal congestion and stuffiness have worsened, as well as how long they have used the nasal decongestant. Treatment of this condition involves stopping the nasal decongestant.

Angioedema

Angioedema is a condition that results in swelling under the skin (**FIGURE 6-8**). The swelling typically occurs in the eyelids, lips, and tongue, but can also affect the gastrointestinal tract and other areas of the body. Angioedema can be hereditary or idiopathic, related to disease or allergy. It also can be an adverse effect of certain medications. Drug-induced angioedema has been reported with use of angiotensin-converting enzyme (ACE) inhibitors and nonsteroidal anti-inflammatory agents (Fine, 1993; Kaplan, 2005; Kulthanan, 2007; Leeyaphan, 2010; Vleeming, 1998). Angioedema can appear shortly after the initiation of drug therapy or after long-term use of the causative agent. Because this adverse effect involves swelling that could potentially compromise breathing, patients should be advised to stop the agent and seek further medical treatment with the primary care provider or emergency treatment if they are experiencing breathing difficulties (Vleeming, 1998). A pharmacist's assessment of possible drug-induced angioedema should include questions that would help determine a time relationship between the development of symptoms and the start of suspected medications. Because angioedema is also seen in

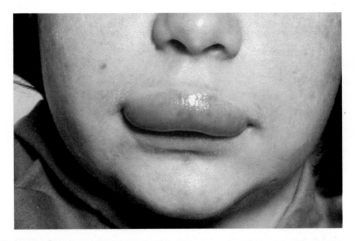

FIGURE 6-8 Angioedema.
© Wellcome Image Library/Custom Medical Stock Photo

allergic reactions, questions related to the presence of urticaria or hives, or other types of rashes should be included (Kaplan, 2005).

Candidiasis

Oral candidiasis is an infection due to the overgrowth of the *Candida* fungus in the mouth cavity (Gonsalves, 2007). Pseudomembranous candidiasis, also known as thrush, appears as white patches in the mouth that can be easily scraped off. Medications, including inhaled corticosteroids, broad spectrum antibiotics, immunosuppressant agents, and chemotherapy can cause thrush. Treatment of this condition requires topical or systemic antifungals, and therefore would warrant referral to a physician (Akpan, 2002; Scully, 2000; Gonsalves, 2007). Pharmacists can play a role in the prevention of oral candidiasis in patients using inhaled corticosteroids by reminding them to rinse their mouth out after each inhaler use.

Cultural Considerations with the Head, Eyes, Ears, Nose, and Throat Exam

Because most of the patient assessment of the head, eyes, ears, nose, and throat involves interviewing the patient, utilizing interview techniques and questions that involve an explanatory model would be helpful in understanding the patient's point of view on how they believe the condition started and how they believe it should be treated. As an example, a study by Klonoff and Landrine (1994) reported that people who believe that the cause of a headache was emotional were more likely to treat the headache using self-care measures rather than seeking medical help. In the case of a patient who presents with headaches, the pharmacist, using an explanatory model, can help determine if the patient believes that the underlying cause of the headache is emotional while continuing to assess the patient to make sure that the headache can be treated using self-care measures. If, during the assessment, the pharmacist discovers that the headache may be a symptom of an underlying condition, proper referral options can then be discussed with the patient.

Using an explanatory model can also help the pharmacist learn about additional causes of headaches specific to various cultures. Foods and beverages such as chocolate, cheese, spicy foods, fruit, tea, and alcohol have been reported to cause headaches in people of various cultures (D'Alessandro, 1988; Gibb, 1991). In addition, other factors such as sun exposure and wearing headdresses or head scarves have been implicated. Although these elements have been studied across different cultures, the incidence of these agents causing a headache is not the same across cultures (Tan, 1997). Therefore, persons from one culture may not develop a headache due to heat and therefore may not identify heat as a cause of headache, whereas persons from another culture may readily attribute heat as a causative factor for headache (D'Alessandro, 1988; Hanifah, 1994).

Another cultural element pharmacists should be aware of is the prevalence and risk of developing certain conditions in various ethnic groups. For example, ACE inhibitor–induced angioedema has a high incidence in African Americans (Brown, 1996). Thus, a pharmacist not only could counsel the African American patient on this adverse effect, but also should have a more acute awareness of this adverse effect if an African American patient presents with symptoms suggestive of angioedema while taking an ACE inhibitor.

Children from low socioeconomic backgrounds and children who attend daycare are at a higher risk of developing otitis media (Zhang, 2014; Uhari, 1996). When a pharmacist is aware of these risk factors, he or she will be able to not only provide valuable education to the parent or patient, but also help to ensure the patient receives prompt care if the symptoms do arise.

Summary

Common disorders of the head and neck can be assessed by the pharmacist by performing a patient interview. Valuable information can be obtained with the use of core questions related to onset, location, duration, character, aggravating factors, relieving factors, timing, and severity of the problem. This information can help the pharmacist determine if the problem can be treated with or without further medical care. In addition, as drug experts, pharmacists can utilize skills to help identify drug-related causes of conditions that can affect the head and neck. Last, with the use of explanatory models during the patient interview, pharmacists can learn more about the patient's beliefs regarding the development and treatment of certain conditions.

Review Questions

1. FM, a 50-year-old man, approaches you at the pharmacy for a recommendation for his "bad hay fever." During your interview of FM, he explains to you that he has been using a nasal decongestant spray that contains oxymetazoline for the past 2 weeks; however, he has noticed that for the past 3 or 4 days the spray is not working as well as it used to. He states that he believes his nose is more congested and stuffy than before. Based on your assessment, what is the most likely cause of FM's worsening symptoms?

2. What questions could one ask to differentiate among a canker sore, a cold sore, and oral candidiasis?

References

Brown NJ, Ray WA, Snowden M, et al. Black Americans have an increased rate of angiotensin converting enzyme inhibitor-associated angioedema. *Clin Pharmacol Ther.* 1996;60:8–13.

Brozek J, Bousquet J, Baena-Cagnani C, Bonini S, Canonica G, Casale T, et al. Allergic rhinitis and its impact on asthma (ARIA) 2010 revision. http://www.whiar.org/docs/ARIAReport_2010.pdf. Accessed July 26, 2014.

Gibbs C, Lip G, Beevers D. Angioedema due to ACE inhibitors: increased risk in patients of African origin. *Br J Clin Pharmacol.* 48, 861–865.

Kaplan AP, Greaves MW. Angioedema. *J Am Acad Dermatol.* 2005;53:373–388.

Leiberthal A, Carroll A, Chonmaitree T, Ganiats T, Hoberman A, Jackson M, et al. The diagnosis and management of acute otitis media. *Pediatrics.* 2013;131(3):e964–e999.

Ramey JT, Bailen E, Lockey RF. Rhinitis medicamentosa. *J Investig Allergol Clin Immunol.* 2006;16(3):148–155.

Rietveld RP, ter Riet G, Bindels PJ, Sloos JH, van Weert HC. Predicting bacterial cause in infectious conjunctivitis: cohort study on informativeness of combinations of signs and symptoms. *BMJ.* 2004;329:206–210.

Rospond RM. Eyes and Ears. In: Jones R, Rospond R., eds. *Patient Assessment in Pharmacy Practice.* Philadelphia, PA: Lippincott Williams & Wilkins; 2003:129–156.

Scolaro KL. Disorders related to colds and allergy. In: Berardi R, Kroon LA, McDermott JH, Newton GD, Oszko MA, Popovich N, et al., eds. *Handbook of Nonprescription Drugs: An Interactive Approach to Self-Care.* 15th ed. Washington, DC: American Pharmacists Association; 2009:201–228.

Uhari M, Mantysaari K, Niemeli M. A meta-analytic review of the risk factors for acute otitis media. *CID.* 1996;22:1079–1083.

Usatine R, Tinitigan R. Nongenital herpes simplex virus. *Am Fam Physician.* 2010; 82(9):1075–1082.

Vleeming W, Van Amsterdam J, Strickler B, de Wildt D. ACE inhibitor-induced angioedema incidence, prevention, and management. *Drug Safety.* 1998;18(3):171–188.

Zhang Y, Xu M, Zhang J, Zeng L, Wang Y, Zheng Q. Risk factors for chronic and recurrent otitis media–a meta-analysis. *PLoS ONE.* 2014;9(1):e86397.doi:10.1371/journal.pone.0086397.

Chapter 7

Cardiovascular Assessment

Antoine T. Jenkins, PharmD, BCPS
Janene L. Marshall, PharmD, BCPS

LEARNING OBJECTIVES

At the completion of this chapter, the reader should be able to:

1. Determine the appropriate questions to ask patients when performing a focused cardiovascular patient interview.
2. Explain the clinical presentation of common cardiovascular diseases.
3. Explain how the clinical presentation of common cardiovascular diseases can differ among various cultures.
4. Explain how to correctly perform the physical assessment techniques related to the cardiovascular system.
5. List medications that can cause adverse effects or medical conditions affecting the cardiovascular system.
6. Explain the clinical presentation of drug-induced disease processes.
7. Triage patients based on clinical presentation of problems related to the cardiovascular system.
8. Explain the varying cultural perspectives on healthcare-seeking behavior.

KEY TERMS

Angina pectoris

Ausculatory gap

Auscultation

Blood pressure

Bradycardia

Diastole

Heart rate (HR)

Heart sounds

Hypertension

Ischemic heart disease (IHD)

Korotkoff sounds

Murmers

Myocardial infarction

Palpate

Systole

Tachycardia

© ontishock/Shutterstock, Inc.

Introduction

The morbidity associated with cardiovascular disease (CVD) has had a substantial impact on individuals living in the United States. One in every three Americans has hypertension, with many not even aware that they have it (Roger, 2012). In modern times, conditions that were once believed to affect only adults, such as dyslipidemia, now plague many adolescents, further extending the widespread presence of this disease. For decades, CVD has been the number one cause of mortality in the United States (Daniels, 2008). Nearly 2,300 Americans die daily, averaging one death every 38 seconds (Roger, 2012). Additionally, CVD claims more lives annually than cancer, pulmonary diseases, and accidents combined (Roger, 2012). Inhabitants of industrialized countries are heavily exposed to elements that can easily prompt the development of the risk factors that ultimately result in CVD. Moreover, specific populations of patients may be disproportionately affected more than others. Because of the widespread presence of this condition, healthcare providers need to be adequately prepared to provide optimum care for these patients. Pharmacists play a significant role in the management of CVD. Because of our availability, patients have easy access to the multitude of services that pharmacists are able to render.

Components of the Cardiovascular System

Heart Sounds

Heart sounds:
The sound produced by the heart during the cardiac cycle.

The cardiac cycle is a repeating series of contractions and relaxations of the cardiac muscle that moves blood through the heart. **Heart sounds** are the hallmark sounds heard during the cycle, "lub-dub," that represent valvular closure. This cycle is composed of two phases:

Systole:
Period of ventricular contraction. The blood is ejected from the heart out into systemic and pulmonic circulation.

1. **Systole**, which represents the period of ventricular contraction. During this phase, blood is ejected from the heart out into systemic and pulmonic circulation. Elevated pressure within the ventricles causes both the tricuspid and the mitral valves to close, resulting in the first heart sound (S_1), or the "lub" sound (Seely, 2000). This sound is best heard over the heart's apex (bottom of the heart located at the fifth intercostal space at the midclavicular line).

Diastole:
Relaxation of the ventricles. During this period, blood is supplied to the heart muscle itself.

2. **Diastole**, which represents relaxation of the ventricles. During this period, blood is supplied to the heart muscle itself. As the ventricles fill with blood, pressure falls within the chambers, causing the aortic and pulmonic valves to close, resulting in the second heart sound (S_2), or the "dub" sound (Seely, 2000). This sound is loudest at the base of the heart (top of the heart located at the second intercostal space to the right and left of the sternum). S_1 and S_2 are sounds of a normal functioning adult heart.

The Physical Exam

Evaluating heart sounds is not within a pharmacist's usual scope of practice; however, it is important to have a complete understanding of abnormalities found upon physical assessment in order to provide the best care for the patient. There are additional heart sounds, S_3 and S_4, that could be indicative of an underlying cardiac condition. Both of these sounds are low-pitched and occur because of blood rapidly rushing from an atrium into a stiffened ventricle. Both are audible at the heart's apex (Swartz, 2002). S_3 can be detected immediately after S_2.

This can be a normal finding in healthy children and young adults; however, in older individuals, the presence of this sound is associated with acute heart failure or hypervolemia. S_4 occurs just prior to ventricular contraction, which is prior to S_1, and can be detected in those with **ischemic heart disease (IHD)** or aortic stenosis. Other sounds include **murmurs**, which are vibrations resulting from turbulent blood flow within the heart chambers or across the valves. They are classified in multiple ways based on location, intensity, and place in the cardiac cycle when they are most detectable. Although the presence of a murmur can be harmless in some individuals, in others they can be suggestive of cardiac disease.

When assessing heart sounds, the surrounding environment should be as quiet as possible. There are four classic auscultatory sites (**FIGURE 7-1**) on the chest where sounds originating at each valve are the most audible (Swartz, 2002). These are the aortic, pulmonic, tricuspid, and mitral areas. There is a fifth location known as Erb's point that is located at the third intercostal space; pulmonic or aortic sounds can also be detected here. When listening to these areas, the examiner needs to use the diaphragm of the stethoscope, applying firm pressure. S_1 and S_2 should also be assessed with the diaphragm. S_1 is best heard over the apex, whereas S_2 is heard clearest at the base. The examiner should assess for the

Ischemic heart disease (IHD):
A narrowing of the blood vessels that supply oxygen and blood to the heart.

Murmurs:
Vibrations resulting from turbulent blood flow within the heart chambers or across the valves.

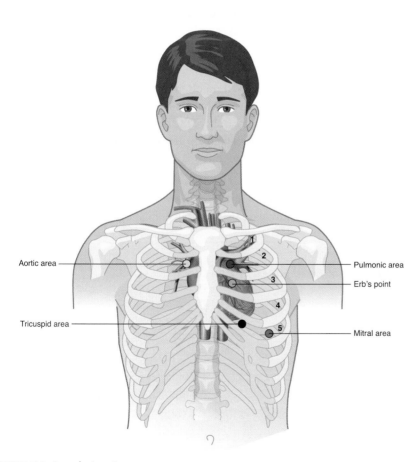

Aortic area

Pulmonic area

Erb's point

Tricuspid area

Mitral area

FIGURE 7-1 Auscultation sites.

presence of S₃ and S₄ by lightly pressing the bell of the stethoscope against the chest. These sounds are detectable over the apex of the heart with the patient lying on his or her left side.

The Patient Interview

Detecting heart sounds can be a difficult skill to master. It requires ample experience for a diagnostician to become proficient. Pharmacists usually have to rely on other clinicians, largely physicians, to make the determination of the presence of an abnormal heart sound. Once an accurate diagnosis is made, the pharmacist can certainly be instrumental in ensuring that evidence-based pharmacotherapy is provided, if necessary, to manage the resulting condition, such as ischemic heart disease. Upon interview, the pharmacist may be able to deduce that a patient could potentially have an abnormal heart sound present. Additionally, patients with a past medical history significant for specific ailments such as congenital heart disease or rheumatic fever are often predisposed to having either a murmur or an abnormal heart sound present. Potential questions that can be posed when making an evaluation include:

- How often do you experience shortness of breath? Swelling in your feet?
- Exactly how would you describe your chest pain? (See the Ischemic Heart Disease section.)
- Has your doctor ever told you that you have a heart murmur?
- Does your heart ever feel as if it is skipping beats?

Heart Rate

Heart rate:
Also known as *pulse*. Measure of the number of contractions or beats per minute (bpm).

As the heart contracts, blood is pushed through the blood vessels. This contraction can cause the blood to pulsate against the vessels and it can be felt among the peripheral vessels. The pulse or **heart rate** (HR) is a measure of the number of contractions or beats per minute (bpm). Normal heart rates for various age groups are listed in **Table 7-1**. A normal heart rate for an adult is 60–100 bpm (Medline, 2013; Jones, 2003).

The Patient Interview

During the patient interview, it is important to investigate potential causes of abnormal heart rates. Both the medication and the social history should be obtained. **Tachycardia**

Tachycardia:
Heart rate is greater than 100 bpm.

Table 7-1 Normal Heart Rates by Age Group

Age	Heart Rate
Birth	90–190 beats per minute
0–6 months	80–180 beats per minute
6–12 months	75–155 beats per minute
1–2 years	70–150 beats per minutes
2–6 years	68–138 beats per minute
6–10 years	65–125 beats per minute
10–14 years	55–115 beats per minute
14 years–adult	60–100 beats per minute

for an adult patient is when the heart rate is greater than 100 bpm. Tachycardia can be caused by stress, excitement, anger, or increased thyroid activity (i.e., hyperthyroidism) or it can be drug-induced by alpha-agonists such as decongestants (e.g., pseudoephedrine), corticosteroids, or nonsteroidal anti-inflammatory drugs (NSAIDs) (Medline, 2013; Hulisz, 2008). The pharmacist could ask if the patient has felt palpitations, light-headed, dizzy, short of breath, or fatigued in order to determine if the patient is experiencing any effects from the elevated heart rate.

Bradycardia is a heart rate less than 60 bpm. A noteworthy clinical finding may be detected with well-trained athletes; they often have a normal resting HR of less than 60 bpm (Mayoclinic, 2013). Bradycardia can also be caused by grief and drug therapy such as beta blockers. During the interview, the pharmacist can ask if the patient tires easily while exercising, feels short of breath or fatigued, or has ever fainted or felt light-headed. Pharmacists should still assess the pulse of patients receiving beta-blocker therapy. If the heart rate is below 50 bpm, especially if the patient is also symptomatic, the patient's drug therapy needs to be assessed and the medication may need to be temporarily discontinued or the dose may need to be decreased.

Bradycardia:
Resting heart rate less than 60 beats per minute.

Pulse Measurement

To measure the radial pulse, do the following:
1. Place the pads of the first and second fingers of your hand on the ventral surface of the patient's wrist medial to the radius bone (**FIGURE 7-2**).
2. Press down until the pulse is felt, but be careful not to occlude the artery, in which case a pulse would not be felt. You should not use your thumb because it has a pulse that can be felt.
3. Count the number of heartbeats in 30 seconds. After 30 seconds, multiply the number by 2. This number will give the beats per minute or the patient's heart rate.

Data from National Institutes of Health. Pulse. Available at: http://www.nlm.nih.gov/medlineplus/ency/article/003399.htm. Accessed April 7, 2013.

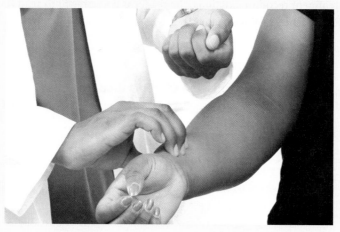

FIGURE 7-2 Pulse measurement.
© val lawless/ShutterStock, Inc.

Case #1

MJ is a 52-year-old woman presenting to your clinic for a follow-up visit regarding her hypertension. Her medication list consists of metoprolol succinate 50 mg by mouth daily, hydrochlorothiazide 25 mg by mouth daily, and Oscal Calcium+D by mouth twice daily. You measure a heart rate of 55 bpm.

Questions

1. Is MJ's heart rate normal, bradycardic, or tachycardic?
2. Are there any possible drug-related causes for MJ's bradycardia?

Palpate:
To examine by touch or feel.

The Physical Exam

In order to determine the heart rate, the peripheral pulse is normally **palpated**, because the artery is very close to the skin at the knees, neck, or wrist. Healthcare professionals most commonly use the radial pulse in order to measure the heart rate.

Blood Pressure

Blood pressure:
Measure of the force of the blood as it is pushed against the arterial walls.

Blood pressure is a measure of the force of the blood as it is pushed against the arterial walls. It is indicative of how hard the heart is working to supply blood from the heart to the major organs in the body and the periphery. Blood pressure consists of two components: systolic pressure and diastolic pressure, as defined in Heart Sounds earlier in this chapter. According to the Seventh Report of the Joint National Committee on Prevention, Detection, Evaluation, and Treatment of High Blood Pressure (JNC 7; Chobanian et al., 2003), blood pressure can be classified in four stages, each outlined in **Table 7-2**. A blood pressure above 140/90 mm Hg is termed **hypertension**. Pharmacists use blood pressure measurements to make adjustments to antihypertensive medications and to assess CVD risk. For specific treatment recommendations, the reader is encouraged to read the guidelines from the JNC 8 panel members (James et al., 2014).

Hypertension:
A blood pressure equal to or above 140/90 mm Hg.

Table 7-2 Blood Pressure Classification

Classification	Systolic (mm Hg)	Diastolic (mm Hg)
Normal	< 120	< 80
Prehypertension	120–139	80–89
Stage 1 hypertension	140–159	90–99
Stage 2 hypertension	≥ 160	≥ 100

*The clinician should use the higher of the two numbers to classify the blood pressure.

Reproduced from Chobanian AV, Bakris GL, Black HR, et al. The seventh report of the Joint National Committee on Prevention, Detection, Evaluation, and Treatment of High Blood Pressure: the JNC 7 report. *JAMA.* 2003;289(19):2560–2572. Epub 2003 May 14.

The Patient Interview

During an interview for an evaluation of blood pressure, the patient's age, ethnic background, and family history of hypertension should be obtained. A thorough medication history should be obtained including prescription, over-the-counter, and herbal medications. The current social history should also be obtained from the patient, including diet and exercise regimen and smoking status. The following factors can cause increased blood pressure readings (Jones, 2003; Perloff, 1993):

- *Age:* Blood pressure increases as the patient matures.
- *Race:* Hypertension occurs more often in minority groups such as African Americans than in Caucasians.
- *Time of day:* Blood pressure is lowest in the early morning and highest during the late afternoon and early evening.
- *Body weight:* Increases in body weight can cause elevations in blood pressure.
- *Emotions:* Fear, anxiety, or stress, as well as pain, can cause increases.
- *Drug-induced causes:* Decongestants (e.g., pseudoephedrine), nonsteroidal anti-inflammatory drugs (NSAIDs; e.g., ibuprofen), and corticosteroids (e.g., prednisone) have been shown to increase blood pressure.

The clinician should be aware of these factors in the assessment of the patient's blood pressure. The clinician should ask if the patient drank any coffee or soda that day, when the patient last smoked a cigarette, and if their bladder is empty. If the patient has consumed caffeine, you should wait 30 minutes before taking the blood pressure. Each cigarette the patient smokes can cause a temporary increase in blood pressure because nicotine is a vasoconstrictor (O'Brien, 2003; Perloff, 1993). As stated previously, these are factors the clinician should be aware of that can cause an increase in the blood pressure reading.

Case #1 *(continued)*

MJ returns to your clinic 4 weeks later for a follow-up visit. During your interview you discover that she has a cold and has been taking pseudoephedrine for the past 3 days. You also note that she has been taking over-the-counter ibuprofen for knee pain caused by gardening.

Question
3. State all the possible risk factors for an increased blood pressure for MJ for today's visit.

The Physical Exam

Two methods can be used to measure blood pressure. First is a direct method using an intra-arterial catheter, which may be done in critically ill patients. An intra-arterial catheter allows for the direct, continuous measurement of blood pressure by inserting a catheter into an artery, such as the radial or femoral artery. Because this particular technique is invasive, it is generally reserved for the critically ill. Blood pressure is most commonly measured indirectly using a stethoscope and sphygmomanometer (Perloff, 1993) (**FIGURE 7-3**). Due to their availability and convenience, patients, as well as outpatient physician offices, may use an electronic blood pressure monitor in place of a manual device. Electronic/digital cuffs are available as arm monitors and wrist monitors (Skirton, 2011) (**FIGURES 7-4** and **7-5**). There are advantages and disadvantages to manual and electronic monitors. See **Tables 7-3** and **7-4**.

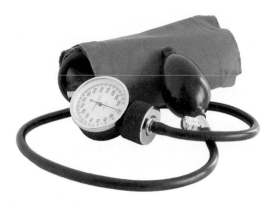

FIGURE 7-3 Blood pressure cuff.
© Donna Beeler/ShutterStock, Inc.

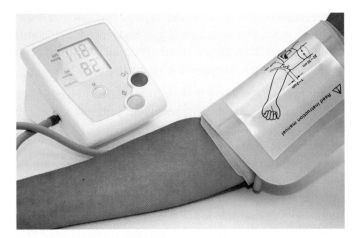

FIGURE 7-4 Digital arm blood pressure monitor.
© Paul Maguire/ShutterStock, Inc.

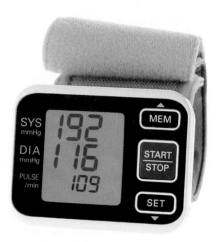

FIGURE 7-5 Digital wrist blood pressure monitor.
© iStockphoto/Thinkstock

Table 7-3 Pros and Cons of Electronic/Digital Monitors

Pros	Cons
Easier to read	An inaccurate reading can be obtained by body position or irregular heart rate.
Inflation automatic (most devices)	Some models are expensive.
Deflation automatic	
Good for the hearing impaired to use	

Table 7-4 Pros and Cons of Manual Blood Pressure Measurement

Pro	Cons
More accurate	Can be cumbersome to use with only one person
	Can be difficult to hear Korotkoff sounds

As the blood flows through the arteries, it produces **Korotkoff sounds**, which occur in five phases (**Table 7-5**). Clinicians manually measure blood pressure by **auscultation**, or listening to the Korotkoff sounds with a stethoscope, in order to identify the systolic and diastolic blood pressures.

Korotkoff sounds: Arterial sounds heard when a stethoscope is applied to the brachial artery and pressure is applied from a sphygmomanometer in order to determine the systolic and diastolic blood pressure.

Table 7-5 Korotkoff Sounds

Phase	Sound	Application
Phase I	First clear tapping sound, may be faint or strong	Initial flow of blood resumes through brachial artery; this is the systolic reading
Phase II	Softer swishing or murmur sound	Undetermined
Phase III	Louder, crisp beat	Undetermined
Phase IV	Sound changes from crisp/clear to muffled	First level of diastolic pressure; useful in exercise assessment
Phase V	Sounds cease (last audible sound)	Circulation no longer audible; this is the diastolic reading

Data from Pickering T, Hall J, Appel L, et al. Recommendations for blood pressure measurement in humans and experimental animals. Part I. Blood pressure in humans. A statement for professionals from the Subcommittee of Professional and Public Education of the American Heart Association on High Blood Pressure Research. *Circulation*. 2005;111:697-716.

Auscultation: The act of listening to the sounds made by the internal organs with or without a stethoscope, in order to aid in the diagnosis or classification of certain disorders.

Common Errors

Several factors can cause an inaccurate measurement. First, the appropriate size cuff should be obtained. The cuff will have an index line marking (Figure 7-6) that indicates if the circumference of the patient's arm fits inside the range area of the cuff. The circumference of a regular adult cuff is typically 27–34 centimeters (cm). For pediatric patients a smaller pediatric cuff should be used, which fits an arm circumference of 18–26 cm. For obese patients an extra-large cuff should be used, which is typically 35–44 cm. Using a cuff that is too small can lead to falsely high readings; using a cuff that is too large can lead to falsely low readings. Stress, anxiety, excitement, or pain can cause increased blood pressure readings. Having a patient empty his or her bladder prior to obtaining a reading could be helpful. Some patients may experience a phenomenon called *white coat syndrome* in which patients experience an increase in blood pressure when it is taken by a clinician, but at home the patients have normal blood pressure values (Perloff, 1993). Also, deflating the cuff too quickly can cause a falsely low systolic and/or a falsely high diastolic reading.

The elderly can experience an **auscultatory gap** when a blood pressure reading is taken. An auscultatory gap is a lengthy disappearance of Korotkoff sounds between phase I and phase V. Initially, the clinician measuring the blood pressure manually will hear tapping sounds; those sounds will disappear for a length of time and then reappear. It can cause an underestimation of the systolic blood pressure and at times an overestimation

---

Auscultatory gap: When assessing blood pressure, the lengthy disappearance of Korotkoff sounds between phase I and phase V.

Blood Pressure Measurement

For accurate measurement of blood pressure, follow these steps:

1. Select a cuff that is the appropriate size (pediatric, adult, or large). The circumference of the patient's arm should fit inside the index line (**FIGURE 7-6**).
2. The patient should be seated and resting for at least 5 minutes prior to taking blood pressure, to ensure that the patient's heart rate and blood pressure have returned to their baseline values. The patient should be sitting in a chair with their back supported and their arm bared at heart rate level.
3. The patient should not have consumed caffeinated products or smoked at least 30 minutes prior to blood pressure measurement.

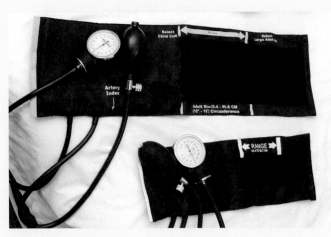

FIGURE 7-6 Blood pressure cuff with index line.

4. Place the cuff on the right or left arm of the patient.
5. The patient and the clinician should not speak while obtaining the blood pressure. The patient talking can cause an increase in the blood pressure reading and it also makes it more difficult for the clinician to hear the Korotkoff sounds.

6. Palpate the brachial artery along the inner upper arm (**FIGURE 7-7**).
7. Place the bladder of the blood pressure cuff over the brachial artery and wrap the cuff snuggly around the arm with the lower edge 1 inch above the antecubital space. Be sure to position the sphygmomanometer in direct line of eyesight.
8. Inflate the cuff 30 mm Hg above the level at which the radial pulse is no longer palpable.
9. Deflate the cuff and wait 30 seconds before reinflating the patient's cuff.

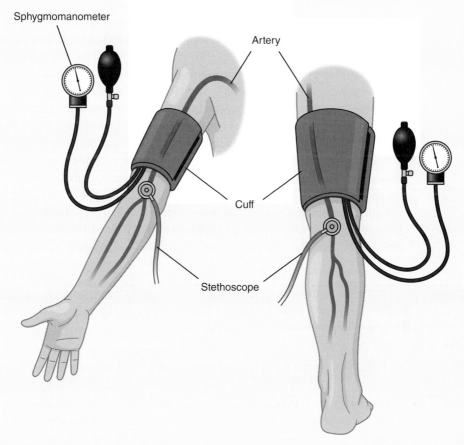

FIGURE 7-7 Stethoscope placement.

Data from Valler-Jones T, Wedgbury K. Measuring blood pressure using the mercury sphygmomanometer. *Br J Nurs*. 2005;14(3):145–150; Jones, R. General assessment and vital signs. In: Jones R, Rospond R, eds. *Patient Assessment in Pharmacy Practice*. Baltimore, MD: Lippincott, Williams & Wilkins; 2003:43–61.

of the diastolic blood pressure. For example, the patient's actual systolic blood pressure is 180 mm Hg with an ausculatory gap from 160–140 mm Hg. The clinician inflates the cuff to 160 mm Hg and does not hear Korotkoff sounds until 140 mm Hg is reached, giving a false systolic blood pressure of 140 mm Hg. Also, if the cuff is inflated to 180 mm Hg, the diastolic blood pressure could be misinterpreted as 160 mm Hg, because this is the start of the ausculatory gap. It is thought to be due to increased arterial stiffness and atherosclerosis in the elderly (Prissant, 2005). It is very important to take a radial blood pressure measurement in this patient population. The pulse at the radial artery should be palpated (Figure 7-2) and the blood pressure cuff inflated until the radial pulse is no longer felt and the pressure is noted. The cuff should be inflated 20–40 mm Hg above the pressure at which the radial pulse was no longer palpated (Smulyan, 2011). This will help to ensure a more accurate blood pressure measurement is taken in this patient population.

Interpretation of Blood Pressure Results and Triage

Pharmacists cannot diagnose hypertension, but should be aware of the clinical guidelines to help manage and triage patients appropriately. Practice guidelines provide recommendations that clinicians can follow for management of blood pressure. If the patient presents to their physician with normal blood pressure, then it should be measured again in 2 years. Patients presenting with prehypertension (Table 7-2) should be rechecked by their primary care physician in 1 year and implement lifestyle modifications such as diet and exercise. If presenting with stage 1 hypertension, the physician may initiate drug therapy and the blood pressure should be reassessed in 2 months. If the patient is presenting to a community pharmacy with previously undiagnosed stage 1 hypertension, the pharmacist should refer the patient to their physician for further follow-up. If the patient was referred to the pharmacist by the physician to manage the hypertension, appropriate medication should be initiated or titrated according to a protocol agreed upon by the pharmacist and physician. If the patient is experiencing a hypertensive urgency, defined as a blood pressure greater than 180/110 mm Hg without acute end organ damage (e.g., **myocardial infarction**, stroke, or renal failure), the pharmacist should refer the patient to their physician for management and the patient should be reevaluated in 1 week. If the patient is experiencing a hypertensive emergency, defined as a blood pressure greater than 180/110 mm Hg with acute end organ damage such as a myocardial infarction or stroke, the patient should be sent to the nearest emergency department (Chobanian, 2003).

> **Myocardial infarction:** Occurs when a blood clot has blocked one of the arteries of the heart causing tissue damage.

Case #1 *(continued)*

You also measure MJ's blood pressure twice (once in each arm) during this patient visit. You obtain approximately the same value, 150/82 mm Hg.

Question
  4. How would you classify MJ's blood pressure?

Ischemic Heart Disease

The central tenet of ischemic heart disease (IHD), also known as coronary heart disease and coronary artery disease, involves an imbalance between myocardial oxygen supply and demand. Approximately 18 million Americans age 20 years or older have IHD (Roger, 2012). The most common cause is atherosclerotic plaque accumulation in one of the epicardial coronary arteries. This narrowing of the arteries results in ischemia, a reduction of blood flow to the heart muscle. Patients may have asymptomatic disease; however, when ≥ 70% of the arterial lumen becomes obstructed, individuals may develop **angina pectoris** (angina), discomfort in the chest or adjacent areas due to compromised blood supply to the heart (Trujillo, 2013). A serious complication related to IHD is acute

> **Angina pectoris:** Discomfort in the chest or adjacent areas due to compromised blood supply to the heart. Also known as angina.

coronary syndrome (ACS), a spectrum of diseases that occurs due to rupture or erosion of an atherosclerotic plaque with subsequent thrombosis formation. These patients will have chest pain even while resting. Specific types of angina and the components of ACS are explained in **Table 7-6**.

Clinical Presentation

The trademark symptom of angina is chest discomfort that has the potential to radiate to adjacent areas such as the shoulder or jaw. Chest pain may be described as increased pressure, heaviness, or tightness. Accompanying symptoms may include gastrointestinal complaints such as nausea, vomiting, or excessive belching; others may include dyspnea (shortness of breath), fatigue, dizziness, diaphoresis (excessive sweating), and a sense of impending doom. Pain that is reproducible upon palpation or described as "sharp" with

Table 7-6 Definitions of Anginal Types and Acute Coronary Syndrome

Types of Angina	
Type	Description
Chronic stable angina	Predictable occurrence of chest discomfort resulting from increased physical activity or emotional stress. It is relieved either by resting or by the administration of nitroglycerin.
Variant angina (or Prinzmetal's angina)	Occurs due to vasospasm of the coronary artery at the site of an atherosclerotic plaque; however, the majority of patients will present without significant arterial obstruction. Chest discomfort occurs at rest. Younger individuals may present with this type of angina.
Acute Coronary Syndrome	
Component	Description
Unstable angina	Partial obstruction of the coronary artery. Chest pain has a longer duration, frequency, and severity compared to chronic stable angina. Because cardiac biomarkers are not released, heart muscle is not damaged. Noticeable ECG changes may or may not be present.
Non-ST-segment elevation myocardial infarction	Partial obstruction of the coronary artery. Chest pain has a longer duration, frequency, and severity compared to chronic stable angina. Cardiac biomarkers are released, indicating heart muscle damage. Either commonly identifiable or nonspecific ECG changes will be present.
ST-segment elevation myocardial infarction	Total obstruction of the coronary artery. Chest pain has a longer duration, frequency, and severity compared to chronic stable angina. Cardiac biomarkers are released, indicating heart muscle damage. Elevation of the ST-segment portion of the ECG will be present.

ECG, Electrocardiogram

Data from Didomenico RJ, Cavallari LH. Chronic stable angina. In: Crouch MA, ed. *Cardiovascular Pharmacotherapy: A Point-of-Care Guide*. Bethesda, MD: ASHP; 2010:121–142; Dobesh PP. Acute coronary syndrome. In: Crouch MA, ed. *Cardiovascular Pharmacotherapy: A Point-of-Care Guide*. Bethesda, MD: ASHP; 2010:143–167.

alterations in severity due to inspiration is likely not ischemic chest pain; an alternative diagnosis should be considered.

Some patients may not report major symptoms; they may complain only of the associated symptoms. For example, a patient may claim to have only shortness of breath, diaphoresis, and isolated back pain. Others may experience pain limited to the jaw or shoulder, sleep disturbances, indigestion, or anxiety. Additionally, these symptoms may occur days or even several weeks prior to the index event (known as prodromal symptoms) (McSweeney, 2001). There are even some patients who may not describe any pain at all. This is denoted as an atypical presentation, and can be very misleading not only for the patient, but also for the diagnosing clinician. These symptoms are nonspecific in nature and can mimic other medical conditions, thus potentially leading to an incorrectly presumed problem (by the patient) or an improper diagnosis (by a physician). Patients with diabetes, women, and elderly individuals are most likely to report atypical symptoms. This is not to suggest that these individuals solely present atypically; however, for various reasons, they do have a greater propensity to do so compared to other patient groups.

Diabetes is known to have effects on every organ system in the body. Long-standing disease can result in the development of the microvascular complication of neuropathy. Dysfunction of the autonomic nervous system results in several cardiovascular manifestations such as resting tachycardia and lack of heart rate variability. Additionally, peripheral neuropathy causes diminished pain perception resulting in a higher incidence of silent ischemia (Vinik, 2001).

There are several gender-based differences that may explain why women are more inclined to atypical presentation (Milner, 1999). Females have overall smaller dimensions compared to men with smaller coronary arteries; thus, reductions in the luminal diameter can have a dramatic effect on blood flow (Mosca, 2011). Furthermore, these smaller-sized arteries are more prone to develop endothelial dysfunction, primarily resulting from diminished production of the smooth muscle relaxant, nitric oxide. Thus, the coronary arteries lose the ability to dilate properly. Moreover, women tend to have more diffuse coronary disease with fewer obstructive lesions, whereas men tend to have more localized coronary plaques (Bellasi, 2007).

Finally, reasons for atypical presentation in the elderly are not clearly known; however, several mechanisms have been proposed (Kelly, 2007). For example, changes related to the normal aging process such as attenuated neuronal function (resulting in depressed pain perception) and progressive loss of physiologic reserve have been hypothesized. Altered mental status is a common cause of hospitalization for elderly individuals, and not all causes have a neurologic etiology. Thus, should an older patient present in a confused state, the physician must consider all possible reasons, surprisingly even cardiovascular causes.

Chest pain can be very nonspecific. It is important for the clinician to understand that not all chest pain is due to obstructed blood flow. In fact, not all cardiac causes of chest pain indicate ischemia. Patients may not fully communicate the precise type of discomfort they are experiencing, or they may describe their pain in a manner that requires further clarification. Consequently, obtaining a complete, yet rapid, history is important in order to rule in or out cardiac causes. A thorough physical examination should be performed as well. **Table 7-7** outlines other etiologies related to chest pain.

Table 7-7 Other Potential Causes of Chest Pain

Cardiac	Aortic dissection, pericarditis, myocarditis
Pulmonary	Pulmonary embolism, pneumothrorax, pulmonary hypertension, pleuritis, pneumonia, acute chest syndrome in patients with sickle cell disease
Gastrointestinal	GERD, PUD, gastritis, esophageal rupture, biliary tract disease, pancreatitis, esophageal spasm
Musculoskeletal	Costochrondritis, rib fractures, sternoclavicular arthritis
Dermatologic	Herpes zoster
Psychiatric	Anxiety, depression

*GERD, gastroesophageal reflux disease; PUD, peptic ulcer disease

Data from Didomenico RJ, Cavallari LH. Chronic stable angina. In: Crouch MA, ed. *Cardiovascular Pharmacotherapy: A Point-of-Care Guide.* Bethesda, MD: ASHP; 2010:121–142; and Fihn, SD. et al. 2012. ACCF/AHA/ACP/AATS/ PCNA/SCAI/STS Guideline for the diagnosis and management of patients with stable ischemic heart disease. *Circulation.* 2012; 126:e354–e371.

The Patient Interview

The mnemonic PQRST can be utilized to characterize the chest pain a patient is experiencing. PQRST has been the traditional memory tool used in medicine to assess chest pain and remember the core questions. **Table 7-8** illustrates the components of the assessment tool and the questions that could be posed to a patient.

Table 7-8 PQRST Questions Used to Characterize Chest Pain

Mnemonic Component	Potential Interview Question	Possible Response
Precipitating factors	What makes the pain worse?	Increased physical exertion, emotional stress, cold weather, walking after a large meal, walking against the wind
Palliative factors	What makes the pain better?	Resting, taking nitroglycerin tabs
Quality	How would you describe the pain?	Pressure, tightness, crushing, burning sensation
Region	Where does it hurt?	Epigastric, substernal, scapular, lateral
Radiation	Do you feel bad anywhere else?	Shoulder, jaw, back, arms, abdomen
Severity	On a scale of 1 to 10, with 10 being the worst pain that you have ever felt, how would you rate the pain?	Scale from 1–10. Pain severity is not an indicator of degree of disease. For example, just because a patient rates his or her pain a 9 out of 10 does not mean there is 100% arterial blockage.
Timing	How long does the pain last?	Abruptness of onset. Lasting anywhere from 30 seconds to 5 minutes.

Data from Fihn SD, Gardin JM, Abrams J, et al. 2012 ACCF/AHA/ACP/AATS/PCNA/SCAI/STS guideline for the diagnosis and management of patients with stable ischemic heart disease: a report of the American College of Cardiology Foundation/American Heart Association Task Force on Practice Guidelines, and the American College of Physicians, American Association for Thoracic Surgery, Preventive Cardiovascular Nurses Association, Society for Cardiovascular Angiography and Interventions, and Society of Thoracic Surgeons. *Circulation.* 2012;126:e354–e471.

Case #2

TJ is a 55-year-old man who wants your recommen-dation for something to relieve his "chest irritation"; he is thinking that he has been suffering from bad heartburn. He has been a patron of your pharmacy for many years, and you are familiar with his medical history. You know he is very compliant when it comes to taking his medications. He has chronic stable angina, hypertension, and diabetes. He is looking for some Tums, but would like to know if there is something "better" that you could suggest.

Question

1. He reports that his chest is "irritated." How would you attain clarification of that description? (See **Table 7-9**.)

Clinical judgment may lead you to ask more ques-tions in order to gain further information. The pharmacist should not feel restricted to merely the core questions; others may be asked in order to help with the assessment.

Pharmacist: "Tell me about how long you have been feeling this."

TJ: "For about a few days."

Pharmacist: "What other symptoms do you feel other than the squeezing?"

TJ: "I have been more sweaty and feeling dizzy."

Pharmacist: "I would like to have you check your blood pressure Mr. J. May I have you step over to the machine?

Question

2. Do you think TJ can manage his own symptoms without seeing a physician, or does he ultimately require a referral?

Table 7-9 Applying the PQRST Mnemonic to Characterize TJ's Chest Pain

Mnemonic Component	Potential Interview Question	Anticipated Response
Precipitating factors	What makes the pain worse?	"Nothing really makes it worse, but I have noticed the feeling when I am resting lately."
Palliative factors	What makes the pain better?	"It goes away after a while. This morning I took a nitro tab, and it seems to have worked, but I don't want to use my nitro for heartburn."
Quality	How would you describe the pain?	"Feels like something is squeezing my chest."
Region	Where does it hurt?	"In the middle of my chest."
Radiation	Do you feel bad anywhere else?	"It moves to my throat and face."
Severity	On a scale of 1 to 10, with 10 being the worst pain that you have ever felt, how would you rate the pain?	"Sometimes a 3, other times a 5."
Timing	How long does the pain last?	"About 20 minutes."

Data from Fihn SD, Gardin JM, Abrams J, et al. 2012 ACCF/AHA/ACP/AATS/PCNA/SCAI/STS guideline for the diagnosis and management of patients with stable ischemic heart disease: a report of the American College of Cardiology Foundation/American Heart Association Task Force on Practice Guidelines, and the American College of Physicians, American Association for Thoracic Surgery, Preventive Cardiovascular Nurses Association, Society for Cardiovascular Angiography and Interventions, and Society of Thoracic Surgeons. *Circulation.* 2012;126:e354–e471.

In addition to the questions in Table 7-8, the pharmacist should also evaluate medication use for appropriateness, because improper usage or nonadherence can be preventable contributors to the chest discomfort. This is especially vital for those patients with a known history of chronic stable angina. Furthermore, questions regarding other issues such as eating habits and social history may be asked in order to gain a complete picture. Patients with known ischemic heart disease and those with no such history can be asked other specific questions to help the clinician determine the source of chest discomfort (see later in this chapter). Allow the patient's responses to the PQRST questions to guide your subsequent questions.

Chest discomfort can be a daunting experience, for both the patient and the clinician. It is understandable for a patient to think that she or he may be having a heart attack when the real issue could be gastroesophageal reflux disease (GERD). For the clinician, because there are multiple causes of chest pain, determining a definitive cause can be difficult, especially for the patient who presents in an atypical fashion. It is strongly advised for any patient who experiences persistent chest pain to immediately seek emergency services. However, there may be some scenarios in which a patient could potentially provide self-care. Thus, should a patient ask for specific recommendations from a pharmacist, he or she needs to completely evaluate each situation prior to determining the best plan of action. Applying clinical judgment is absolutely essential when dealing with chest pain, because an incorrect decision could be potentially life-threatening. The pharmacist must tailor recommendations based on the patient in question. As previously stated, in addition to the PQRST questions, more specific questions may need to be asked in order to obtain a complete history. The pharmacist should also educate individuals on atypical presentations, particularly those susceptible patients with a history of IHD. Refer to **Tables 7-10** and **7-11** for specific scenarios.

Table 7-10 Specific Pharmacist–Patient Communications in Cases of Known History of Chronic Stable Angina

Interview Question	Patient Response	Issue	Decision
Tell me how you take the medications your doctor has prescribed.	"I only take them when I feel bad."	Noncompliance	Self-care: Assess rationale for noncompliance and make recommendations based on what the patient tells you. Explain the role of each medication. If cost is an issue, you may consider contacting the prescriber regarding less expensive alternatives.
Where at home do you keep your nitroglycerin tabs that you place under your tongue?	"In my pill box."	Improper medication storage	Self-care: Patients must be educated on proper storage. These tablets must be kept in the original container in order to maintain potency. They must also be stored at room temperature.

(continues)

Table 7-10 Specific Pharmacist–Patient Communications in Cases of Known History of Chronic Stable Angina (*continued*)

Interview Question	Patient Response	Issue	Decision
When exactly do you take your Isordil (isosorbide dinitrate) or nitroglycerin patch?	Isosorbide dinitrate: "I take one in the morning and one at bedtime." Patch: "I apply one every morning."	Incorrect administration	Self-care: Patients who use nitroglycerin must ensure a nitrate-free interval in order to prevent tolerance. Isosorbide dinitrate should be given at specific times each day in order to provide the appropriate interval. The patch must be removed after 12 hours each day (usually removed at bedtime).
What new medications has your doctor prescribed?*	"I now take Celebrex (celecoxib) for my arthritis."	Drug-induced myocardial ischemia	Pharmacist–prescriber communication: The patient should be informed that celecoxib (a COX-II inhibitor) can cause increases in blood pressure. The patient should inform the physician that they have also been diagnosed with hypertension so the risks versus benefits of continuing with a COX-II inhibitor for pain can be weighed.
What medications are you taking over the counter?*	"I have been using Yohimbine because Viagra (sildenafil) is so expensive."	Drug-induced hypertension	Self-care: Patients must be educated to avoid certain over-the-counter medications because some can provoke an increase in blood pressure. Use of illicit substances such as cocaine should be strongly discouraged.
What makes your pain better?	"Nothing is working. I tried resting and three nitroglycerin tabs."	ACS	Immediate physician referral: Persistent pain unrelieved with usual palliative measures warrants further evaluation. Patients should be educated to call 911 if they get no relief from the first sublingual nitroglycerin tablet.
Have you ever had isolated back or jaw pain?*	"Yes."	Possible atypical presentation	Use best clinical judgment: Atypical presentation of IHD can be extremely deceiving. The pharmacist must educate those patient groups most prone to presenting in this fashion (women, diabetics, and the elderly). Should a patient report these symptoms, further evaluate them. Determine if there are possible causes of back pain (increase in physical activity) or if other symptoms are present, such as dyspnea, nausea, or vomiting. Ask about current medical conditions and social and family history. These symptoms should not be ignored and may warrant referral to a physician.

*Scenario could also occur in those with an unknown history of IHD.

Data from Crouch MA, ed. *Cardiovascular Pharmacotherapy: A Point-of-Care Guide.* Bethesda, MD; American Society of Health-System Pharmacists; 2010.

Table 7-11 Specific Pharmacist–Patient Communications in Cases with Unknown History of Ischemic Heart Disease

Interview Question	Patient Response	Issue	Decision
How would you describe your chest pain?	"I feel increased pressure and tightness when I am doing chores around the house, but it goes away when I am resting."	Chronic stable angina	Further assessment is needed. Physician referral is required.
	"Feels like a burning sensation, usually after I eat a meal."	GERD	Self-care and/or physician referral: Could recommend a trial of antacids and avoidance of certain items such as spicy foods. Physician referral would ultimately be necessary should symptoms persist.
	"It is a sharp pain.... It happened right after I lifted weights a few days ago."	Musculoskeletal	Self-care and/or physician referral: Could recommend use of hot pads or an analgesic. Physician referral would ultimately be necessary should the pain persist.
On a scale of 1–10, with 10 being the worst pain in your life, how would you rate your pain?	"It's a 10."	Various	Although pain is subjective, should a patient describe pain of this magnitude, he or she should seek emergency services immediately.

Data from Crouch MA, ed. *Cardiovascular Pharmacotherapy: A Point-of-Care Guide*. Bethesda, MD; American Society of Health-System Pharmacists; 2010.

Clinical Presentation of Drug-Induced Processes

Because individuals are living longer than those from decades past, the chance of developing a chronic medical condition that requires pharmacotherapy increases.

With an influx of new drugs being introduced to the market, the prevalence of adverse drug events (ADEs) has become more commonplace. Interestingly, postmarketing data has revealed cardiovascular ADEs from the use of several drugs or drug classes (McSweeney, 2011; Meadows, 2013). The pharmacist, being the drug expert, must remain cognizant to drug-induced diseases. After complete investigation and ruling out other causes, if a drug is suspected of being the culprit, the pharmacist needs to have a dialogue with the prescriber, explaining her or his reasoning and devising the best alternative for the patient. The following sections highlight some common drug-induced processes (Yasuda, 2011).

Beta Blockers and Exercise

When patients exercise they often track the amount of exertion on the heart by measuring their pulse. Patients receiving beta-blocker drug therapy for hypertension have a slower heart rate, thus it is not always possible to achieve the target heart rate during exercise. Patients should be educated to obtain approval from their physician prior to initiating an exercise regimen and make frequent self-assessments during exercise to gauge their fatigue (Mayoclinic, 2013).

Beta Blockers and Diabetes

Beta blockers can mask the signs of hypoglycemia in diabetic patients. Beta blockers block the beta receptors in the sympathetic nervous system. One of the signs of hypoglycemia is increased heart rate. Patients should be educated on other signs and symptoms of hypoglycemia, such as shaking, dizziness or lightheadedness, blurred vision, or headache, if they are taking one of these agents (Mayoclinic, 2013).

Cardiovascular Effects from Illicit Drugs and Common Fad Products

Cocaine is a potent alpha-agonist of the sympathetic nervous system. The ingestion of cocaine stimulates the alpha receptors, causing vasoconstriction and an increase in heart rate and blood pressure (Pitts, 1997).

Methamphetamines have become an increasingly popular drug of abuse. Methamphetamines increase catecholamine release in the nervous system causing an increase in heart rate and blood pressure (Kay, 2013).

"Energy drinks" often contain caffeine. Caffeine is a stimulant that causes an increase in blood pressure and heart rate. Most energy drinks contain the caffeine equivalent of two cups of coffee; when consumed in moderation, they should not be a significant health threat for healthy individuals.

Prior to the initiation of drug therapy, a thorough social history should be obtained from the patient. When managing patients for uncontrolled hypertension, the pharmacist should determine if the patient is compliant with their medication and diet changes. If the patient is on appropriate drug therapy and compliant with the pharmacological and nonpharmacological therapy regimen, and the blood pressure goal still is not achieved, the pharmacist should inquire more about the patient's current social history. Illicit drug use or excessive consumption of energy drinks could be a potential source of the uncontrolled blood pressure (Jahangir, 2013).

Corticosteroid-Induced Hypertension

Corticosteroids such as methylprednisolone or prednisone can cause sodium retention. The retention of sodium also causes fluid retention, which can cause an increase in blood pressure. For patients taking short-term, or burst, steroid therapy, their blood pressure will return to normal once the therapy has ended. If patients who are taking long-term steroid therapy—to prevent organ transplant rejection, for example—experience hypertension, it can be managed with diuretic therapy (Ferrari, 2003).

NSAIDs and COX II Inhibitors and Hypertension

NSAIDs and cyclooxygenase (COX) II inhibitors cause dose-related increases in sodium and water retention. They can cause an increase in renal vascular resistance, which decreases renal perfusion, and can prompt the production of vasoconstricting factors that can cause an increase in blood pressure. The risk versus benefit of using NSAIDs or COX II inhibitors for pain management in patients with uncontrolled hypertension should be assessed. It may be best to recommend an alternative pain medication (Valler-Jones, 2005).

Cultural Considerations for Cardiovascular Disease Assessment

In order to fully assess patients for CVD, pharmacists should have a keen awareness of the culture of the patients being treated. By being mindful of their cultural nuances, patients will be placed more at ease, thus ultimately leading to a successful interview. The more comfortable a patient feels, the more apt they are to provide you with all of the information you need. Consequently, pharmacists will be better prepared to provide the most appropriate recommendations. This includes knowing the culture's attitude regarding seeking health care and cultural beliefs regarding illness. Also, in this age of evidence-based medicine, clinicians have realized that there are cultural differences among the medication classes and should keep these in consideration when recommending medications for their patients (Woodard, 2005).

Medication Efficacy

Angiotensin-converting enzyme (ACE) inhibitors are considered a first-line therapy for many disease states such as heart failure, myocardial infarction, and diabetes. Some patients in certain ethnic groups may have lower levels of renin in circulation as compared to other ethnic groups. Due to this, ACE inhibitors and angiotensin receptor blockers (ARBs) are not as efficacious in this patient population; however, the medication classes are still used and should be recommended because the evidence showing prevention of complications is overwhelming. Thus when compelling indications are present, these patients should not be denied therapy. Often, pairing the drug with a diuretic improves efficacy. Healthcare providers should be aware that some cultures might have some unique pharmacogenetic properties, which can lead to the recommendation of a different dose of the drug than commonly used with other ethnicities (Brown, 1996).

Healthcare-Seeking Behavior Based on Ethnicity and Cultural Beliefs

The patient's culture can influence their decision to seek health care. Some patients may have a distrust of healthcare providers and only seek treatment when absolutely necessary (Bailey, 1987). Some may be inclined to use self-care first in order to treat illness or diseases by using natural remedies, such as drinking a teaspoon of vinegar or lemon juice every day to lower blood pressure due to a belief that it will "cleanse" the blood. Often these home remedies have been passed down from generation to generation, becoming engrained within one's personal beliefs. Religion or spirituality may also be a strong factor in the patient's beliefs regarding health, such as the belief that health is in the hands of God and not the healthcare practitioner, and nothing the practitioner will do will change the final outcome if it is God's will.

It is of the utmost importance for the healthcare provider to be aware of and to be sensitive to these cultural beliefs. Many of these ideals have been passed down through the generations and it may be difficult for one to change. Although the clinician has a responsibility to respect people's principles, he or she has an even greater duty to professionally intervene if those beliefs have the potential to elicit harm. Additionally, when

Case #3

JM is a 68-year-old African American woman who has been a long-time patron of your pharmacy. She has a past medical history remarkable for hypertension and osteoarthritis. She asks the technician to speak to the pharmacist, and she states to you, "Hello, I need to get a refill on my 'pressure pills.'"

Pharmacist: "I will be happy to help you. First, let's see exactly which medications you need refilled. . . .

I see that you take two different blood pressure pills. Do you need the 'water pill' refilled or the other one?"

JM: "The other one. Thank you."

Question

1. What lesson in cultural competency should the pharmacist display?

it comes to medications, pharmacists need to carefully explain the significance of why a particular drug was prescribed and to clarify any misconceptions or fears regarding the drug. This must be done in a manner that the patient can clearly comprehend.

Health Disparities Related to Cardiovascular Disease

Cardiovascular health disparities remain a significant health problem. When evaluating the patient's risk factors, their ethnicity should be taken into consideration because certain ethnic groups may be predisposed to an increased number of risk factors, such as hypertension, diabetes, and dyslipidemia, which puts them at a greater risk to develop CVD. Also, clinicians should be trained to recognize the signs and symptoms of CVD, including atypical signs and symptoms. For instance, women continue to be underdiagnosed and undertreated when it comes to CVD, and a likely reason for this is the atypical manner in which they may present. There are reported lower rates of hospitalization and treatment for various ethnic groups due to lack of access to providers, socioeconomic factors, and lack of recognition of symptoms by practitioners (Vinik, 2001; Jones, 2006).

Summary

The pharmacist's role in assessing the cardiovascular system includes performing a patient interview and performing physical assessments such as blood pressure measurement. The patient interview is a method to gather subjective and objective data from the patient, such as the social and medication history. The pharmacist can use the data obtained from the interview and physical assessment for pharmacotherapy recommendations and to help identify drug-related problems. The patient's culture can influence the medication efficacy and their desire to seek health care. The pharmacist should be sure to take into consideration the patient's beliefs regarding cardiovascular disease when providing recommendations for the patient.

Review Questions

1. ST is a 35-year-old man. He has been a marathon runner for the past 15 years and participates in at least five marathons per year. He also participates in decathlons. Would you expect his heart rate to be bradycardic, normal, or tachycardic?

2. A 62-year-old woman comes to your pharmacy and requests that you take her blood pressure. You note that it is 186/120 mm Hg. She is also complaining of nausea and says that for the past few weeks she just "feels off." How would you classify the patient's blood pressure? What recommendation would you make as the pharmacist?

References

Bailey EJ. Sociocultural factors and health care-seeking behavior among black Americans. *J Natl Med Assoc.* 1987;79(4):389–392.

Bellasi A, Raggi P, Merz CNB, et al. New insights into ischemic heart disease in women. *Clevel Clin J Med.* 2007;74(8):585–594.

Brown NJ, Ray WA, Snowden M, Griffin MR. Black Americans have an increased rate of angiotensin converting enzyme inhibitor-associated angioedema. *Clin Pharmacol Ther.* 1996;60(1):8–13.

Chobanian AV, Bakris GL, Black HR, et al. The seventh report of the Joint National Committee on Prevention, Detection, Evaluation, and Treatment of High Blood Pressure: the JNC 7 report. *JAMA.* 2003;289(19):2560–2572. Epub 2003 May 14.

Daniels SR, Greer FR. Lipid screening and cardiovascular health in childhood. *Pediatrics.* 2008;22:198–208.

Didomenico RJ, Cavallari LH. Chronic stable angina. In: Crouch MA, ed. *Cardiovascular Pharmacotherapy: A Point-of-Care Guide.* Bethesda, MD: ASHP; 2010:121–142.

Dobesh PP. Acute coronary syndrome. In: Crouch MA, ed. *Cardiovascular Pharmacotherapy: A Point-of-Care Guide.* Bethesda, MD: ASHP; 2010:143–167.

Ferrari P. Cortisol and the renal handling of electrolytes: role in glucocorticoid-induced hypertension and bone disease. *Best Pract Res Clin Endocrinol Metab.* 2003;17:575–589.

Gibbons RJ, Abrams J, Chatterjee K, et al. ACC/AHA 2002 guideline update for the management of patients with chronic stable angina—summary article: a report of the American College of Cardiology/American Heart Association Task Force on Practice Guidelines (Committee on the Management of Patients with Chronic Stable Angina). *J Am Coll Cardiol.* 2003;41:159–168.

Hulisz D, Lagzdins M. Drug-induced hypertension. *US Pharm.* 2008;33(9):HS11–HS20.

Jahangir E, Yang EH. Blood pressure assessment. Emedicine. Available at: http://emedicine.medscape.com/article/1948157-overview. Accessed March 29, 2013.

James PA, Oparil S, Carter BL, et al. 2014 evidence-based guideline for the management of high blood pressure in adults report from the panel members appointed to the eighth Joint National Committee (JNC 8). *JAMA.* 2014;311(5):507–520. doi:10.1001/jama.2013.28442.

Jones DE, Weaver MT, Grimley D, Appel SJ, Ard J. Health belief model perceptions, knowledge of heart disease, and its risk factors in educated African-American women: an exploration of the relationships of socioeconomic status and age. *J Natl Black Nurses Assoc.* 2006;17(2):13–23.

Jones R. General assessment and vital signs. In: Jones R, Respond R, eds. *Patient Assessment in Pharmacy Practice.* Baltimore, MD: Lippincott, Williams & Wilkins; 2003:43–61.

Kay S, McKetin R. Cardiotoxicity associated with methamphetamine use and signs of cardiovascular pathology among methamphetamine users. Available at: http://ndarc.med.unsw.edu.au/resource/cardiotoxicity-associated-methamphetamine-use-and-signs-cardiovascular-pathology-among. Accessed August 21, 2013.

Kelly BS. Evaluation of the elderly patient with acute chest pain. *Clin Geriatr Med.* 2007;23(2):327–349.

Mayo Clinic. High blood pressure. Available at: http://www.mayoclinic.com/health/beta-blockers/HI00059/NSECTIONGROUP=2. Accessed April 12, 2013.

McSweeney JC, Cody M, Crane PB. Do you know them when you see them? Women's prodromal and acute symptoms of myocardial infarction. *J Cardiovasc Nurs.* 2001;15:26–38.

Meadows M. Why drugs get pulled off the market. *FDA Consum.* 2002;36(3):3.

MedlinePlus. Pulse. Available at: http://www.nlm.nih.gov/medlineplus/ency/article/003399.htm. Accessed April 7, 2013.

Milner KA, Funk M, Richards S, et al. Gender differences in symptom presentation associated with coronary heart disease. *Am J Cardiol.* 1999;84:396–399.

Mosca L, Barrett-Connor E, Kass Wenger N. Sex/gender differences in cardiovascular disease prevention. What a difference a decade makes. *Circulation.* 2011;124:2145–2154. doi: 10.1161/CIRCULATIONAHA.110.968792.

Myers MG, Godwin M, Dawes M, Kiss A, Tobe SW, Grant FC. Conventional versus automated measurement of blood pressure in primary care patients with systolic hypertension: randomised parallel design controlled trial. *BMJ.* 2011;342:d286.

National Institutes of Health. Addressing cardiovascular health in Asian Americans and Pacific Islanders: a background report. January 2000. Available at: http://www.nhlbi.nih.gov/health/prof/heart/other/aapibkgd/aapibkgd.pdf. Accessed April 30, 2013.

O'Brien E. Ambulatory blood pressure measurement is indispensable to good clinical practice. *J Hypertens.* 2003;21(2 Suppl):S11–S18.

Perloff D, Grim C, Flack J, et al. Human blood pressure determination by sphygmomanometry. *Circulation.* 1993;88:2460–2470.

Pitts WR, Lange RA, Cigarroa JE, et al. Cocaine-induced myocardial ischemia and infarction: pathophysiology, recognition, and management. *Prog Cardiovasc Dis.* 1997;40(1):65–76.

Prissant LM. *Hypertension in the Elderly.* Totowa, NJ: Humana Press; 2005.

Roger VL, Go AS, Lloyd-Jones DM, et al. On behalf of the American Heart Association Statistics Committee and Stroke Statistics Subcommittee. Heart disease and stroke statistics—2012 update: a report from the American Heart Association. *Circulation.* 2012;125:e2–e220.

Seely RR, Stephens TD, Tate P. *Anatomy and Physiology.* 5th ed. Boston, MA: McGraw-Hill; 2000.

Skirton H, Chamberlain W, Lawson C, et al. A systematic review of variability and reliability of manual and automated blood pressure readings. *J Clin Nurs.* 2011;20(5–6):602–614.

Smulyan H, Safar ME. Blood pressure measurement: retrospective and prospective views. *Am J Hypertens.* 2011;24(6):628–634. doi: 10.1038/ajh.2011.22. Epub 2011 Feb.

Sowinski KM. Myocardial ischemia and acute coronary syndrome. In: Tisdale JE, Miller DA, eds. *Drug-Induced Diseases: Prevention, Detection, and Management.* 2nd ed. Bethesda, MD. American Society of Health-System Pharmacists; 2010:401–427.

Swartz MH. *Textbook of Physical Diagnosis: History and Examination.* 4th ed. Philadelphia, PA: WB Saunders; 2002.

Trujilo TC, Nolan PE. Chronic stable angina. In: Alldredge BK, Corelli RL, Ernst ME, et al., eds. *Koda-Kimble and Young's Applied Therapeutics: The Clinical Use of Drugs.* 10th ed. Philadelphia, PA: Lippincott Williams & Wilkins; 2013.

Valler-Jones T, Wedgbury K. Measuring blood pressure using the mercury sphygmomanometer. *Br J Nurs.* 2005;14(3):145–150.

Vinik AI, Erbas T. Recognizing and treating diabetic autonomic neuropathy. *Clevel Clin J Med.* 2001;68(11):928–944.

Woodard LD, Hernandez MT, Lees E, Petersen LA. Racial differences in attitudes regarding cardiovascular disease prevention and treatment: a qualitative study. *Patient Educ Couns.* 2005;57(2):225–231.

Yasuda SU, Zhang L, Huang S-M. The role of ethnicity in variability in response to drugs: focus on clinical pharmacology studies. *Clin Pharmacol Ther.* 2008;84(3):417–423. doi: 10.1038/clpt.2008.141.

© antishock/Shutterstock, Inc.

Chapter 8

Pulmonary Assessment
Yolanda M. Hardy, PharmD

LEARNING OBJECTIVES

At the completion of this chapter, the reader should be able to:

1. Determine appropriate questions to ask patients when performing a focused pulmonary patient interview.

2. Explain the clinical presentation of common symptoms and diseases related to the pulmonary system.

3. Explain how to correctly perform the physical assessment techniques related to the pulmonary system.

4. List medications that can cause adverse effects or medical conditions affecting the pulmonary system.

5. Explain the clinical presentation of drug-induced disease processes.

6. Triage patients based on clinical presentation of problems related to the pulmonary system.

7. Explain cultural considerations related to the pulmonary assessment and patient management of asthma.

KEY TERMS

Bradypnea	Hemoptysis	Percussion
Cyanosis	Hyperventilation	Pneumothorax
Dyspnea	Inspection	Tachypnea

Introduction

This chapter will discuss portions of the pulmonary system that are pertinent to the pharmacist. The role of the pharmacist in regard to assessment of the pulmonary system can vary greatly. Assessment of the pulmonary system can help the pharmacist determine proper triage for a patient as well as help to determine the extent of disease control of lung disorders. As an example, a pharmacist working in a community pharmacy setting may use a pulmonary assessment to determine if a cough can be managed with over-the-counter agents. On the other hand, a pharmacist working in a pulmonary clinic may use pulmonary assessment to determine the level of control of a patient with asthma. Much of the pulmonary assessment performed by the pharmacist can be completed by way of patient interview; however, in certain cases, physical examination will provide the pharmacist with more information about the patient's problems or concerns.

The patient interview performed for pulmonary conditions utilizes the core questions related to symptom onset, location, duration, character, aggravating factors, relieving factors, timing, and severity; however, depending on the disease process, more focused questions—which will be discussed further in this chapter—may prove beneficial in gathering information about the patient's condition.

Components of the Pulmonary Exam

Inspection:
Method used in physical assessment that involves looking at a specific body area to assess for abnormalities.

Physical examination typically involves **inspection**, auscultation, palpation, and **percussion** of the chest cavity. The two techniques most pertinent to pharmacists are inspection and auscultation (Bickley, 2009). Inspection involves visually looking at the chest while the patient is breathing. When inspecting a patient, it is important to look for signs of using accessory muscles to breathe. These muscles include the scalene, trapezius, and sternomastoid muscles located in the neck (**FIGURE 8-1**). Use of these muscles is a sign of difficulty breathing (Bickley, 2009).

Percussion:
Method used in physical assessment that involves tapping of a specific body area to assess for abnormalities.

Also, it is important to notice the patient's posture and appearance. Patients who are experiencing severe difficulty breathing may sit in the *tripod position* (**FIGURE 8-2**), in which the patient is hunched over, supporting his or her hands on the knees (Bauldoff, 2012). The patient may breathe through pursed lips. The patient also may appear panicked or irritable.

Inspection can also consist of observing the patient for signs of poor oxygenation. A hallmark sign of poor oxygenation is **cyanosis**, described as a bluish color seen on the skin or mucus membranes. Another sign to look for is confusion or lethargy in the patient that is cyanotic (Jones, 2003). These signs warrant immediate treatment.

Cyanosis:
Bluish or grayish coloring seen on the skin near mucous membranes and extremities as a result of poor oxygenation.

Auscultation involves listening to the lungs via stethoscope. During auscultation of the lungs, one is interested in listening to the flow of air through the lungs (Bickley, 2009).

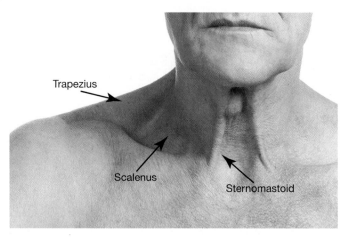

Trapezius

Scalenus

Sternomastoid

FIGURE 8-1 Accessory muscles.
© KyKyPy3HuK/iStock/Thinkstock

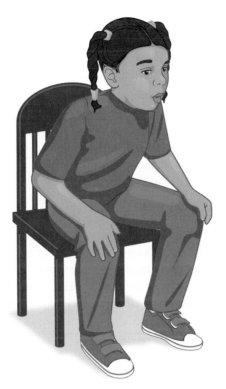

FIGURE 8-2 Tripod position.

Airflow can be altered in patients with lung disease such as asthma, chronic obstructive pulmonary disease (COPD), or cystic fibrosis, or in acute illnesses such as an upper respiratory tract infection.

Palpation involves feeling the chest area to assess for tenderness or abnormalities in chest expansion when the patient is breathing. Percussion involves tapping over the lung area of the chest to determine differences in sound. This will help determine air-filled vs. fluid-filled areas of the chest (Bickley, 2009).

The pulmonary assessment should be employed if a patient complains of difficulty breathing, shortness of breath, chest pain, wheezing, or cough. This assessment should also be employed if the patient has a history of lung disease such as asthma or COPD, or has an acute illness such as an upper respiratory tract infection. Common symptoms as well as common disease states related to the pulmonary system will be discussed in the next section.

Clinical Presentation of Symptoms and Disease Processes Related to the Pulmonary System

Symptoms Related to Respiration

The respiratory rate, or the rate at which a person breathes, can give insight on the patient's lung function. The respiratory rate is defined as the number of breaths a person takes in one minute.

The Patient Interview

In regard to respiratory rate, because patients do not necessarily take note of their breathing pattern, it would be rare for a patient to present stating that they have noticed a change in their breathing rate. As a result, a patient interview may begin as a result of the pharmacist noticing that the patient's breathing pattern is different or as a result of the patient presenting with other symptoms suggestive of respiratory involvement. The pharmacist could bring this to the patient's attention and follow up with a question such as, "Have you noticed any changes in your breathing?" Based on the patient's answer, the pharmacist could ask additional questions using the core questions to gather more information. If the patient's chart is not available to the pharmacist, the pharmacist should verify if the patient has been diagnosed with any pulmonary disorders.

Dyspnea:
Shortness of breath that can indicate breathing difficulties.

Patients will, however, notice if they are experiencing shortness of breath, or **dyspnea**. Utilizing the core questions can help the pharmacist learn more about this complaint. Some patients may have dyspnea only on exertion, so it is important to ask if they experience shortness of breath when walking or exercising versus at rest (Jones, 2003). Patients with heart failure may experience dyspnea when lying down. As a result, many find that sleeping on pillows or sleeping in a reclining chair helps relieve dyspnea. If the patient has a history of heart failure, or if they mention that sleeping propped up on pillows provides relief, a key question to ask is how many pillows are needed to provide relief (Jones, 2003). Asking about sleeping in a reclining chair is also beneficial. If a patient states that the dyspnea is new or has changed from baseline—for example, the heart failure patient is now sleeping on four pillows rather than two—and is accompanied by cyanosis, lethargy, or central nervous system (CNS) changes, then a referral to the primary care provider or emergency care may be warranted.

The Physical Exam

Calculating the respiratory rate is a simple technique that can be performed unbeknownst to the patient. The clinician simply counts the number of respirations while the patient is at rest and not speaking. When measuring the respiratory rate, one breath equals one cycle of inhalation and exhalation. Rather than counting the respiratory rate for the entire minute, one can count the number of breaths for 10 seconds and multiply this number by 6, or count the number of breaths for 15 seconds and multiply the number by 4. If a patient seems to have an irregular breathing pattern, then it is recommended that the respirations be counted for the entire 60 seconds (Jones, 2003). When measuring the respiratory rate, a key skill in obtaining a reliable reading is to be discreet when performing this assessment. If a person is aware that the clinician is watching him or her breathe, he or she may subconsciously alter the breathing pattern. To minimize the chances of this, the assessment is often performed along with checking the pulse as a way to distract the patient. Also, rather than looking directly at the chest, the pharmacist may look at the area of the neck between the chin and collarbone and watch it rise with inhalation and fall with exhalation. If the pharmacist has difficulty assessing the respiratory rate using this method, he or she may stand beside the patient and watch the chest and diaphragm extend during inhalation and contract during exhalation. As a person ages into adulthood, their respiratory rate decreases (**Table 8-1**). Young children typically have a higher respiratory rate (Jones, 2003).

Table 8-1 Normal Respiratory Rate by Age

Age	Range (breaths/min)
Adults and adolescents	12 to 20
Children (1 to 12 years)	15 to 30
Infants	25 to 50

Rapid, shallow breathing that results in a respiratory rate greater than the normal range is referred to as **tachypnea**. Tachypnea can be a sign of lung disease such as asthma, pulmonary embolism, respiratory infections, or heart failure (Bickley, 2009; Jones, 2003). **Hyperventilation**, which is also characterized by an elevated respiratory rate, is not the same as tachypnea. Hyperventilation can typically occur after strenuous exercise or as a result of anxiety or panic. With hyperventilation, the breaths are typically prolonged and deep, rather than shallow (Bickley, 2009).

Slow breathing, in which the respiratory rate is less than the normal range, is called **bradypnea**. Bradypnea can be due to a number of causes, including respiratory depression due to medication use or increased intracranial pressure (Jones, 2003).

An easy assessment for dyspnea that can be performed along with the patient interview is observing whether the patient can speak in full sentences. While the pharmacist is listening to the patient's responses, he or she should observe whether the patient is able to speak in full sentences or needs to stop to take a breath before completing a sentence. In general, a person can speak multiple sentences before taking a breath in conversation. If the person is unable to do this, it is a possible sign of breathing difficulty. In general, the fewer words that can be spoken between breaths, the more difficult it is for the patient to breathe. This assessment is a very easy one to perform, but one should realize that this is not a fail-safe assessment. It is possible for patients to experience breathing difficulties, but still speak full sentences without a problem.

Tachypnea: Classification that describes a breathing rate considered faster than normal.

Hyperventilation: Rapid, prolonged, deep breathing that can result from exercise, anxiety, or panic.

Bradypnea: Classification that describes a breathing rate considered slower than normal.

Symptoms Related to Airflow in the Lung

When something is impeding airflow in the lung, be it mucus, inflammation of the bronchial tree, inflammation of the epiglottis, or a foreign body, changes in the sound of air flowing through the lungs often occur. Normal lung sounds include vesicular, bronchial, and bronchovesicular sounds (**Table 8-2**). Adventitious, or abnormal, lung sounds include wheezes, rales, rhonchi, crackles, and stridor (Bickley, 2009; Jones, 2003) (Table 8-2).

The Patient Interview

Abnormal lung sounds can be the result of an acute or chronic condition. Therefore, it is important to ask questions to try to determine if the symptoms are of new onset, if the patient has a history of lung disease, and if the patient is experiencing other symptoms in addition to the abnormal lung sounds. Examples of other symptoms include shortness of breath, chest pain, fever, or coughing. These signs and symptoms may be suggestive of other medical conditions, such as pneumonia, pulmonary embolism, heart failure, asthma, or COPD. Because these conditions require further management, a referral to the primary care provider or immediate medical treatment would be warranted.

Table 8-2 Description of Normal and Abnormal Lung Sounds

Bronchial	**Location of sound**	Trachea and larynx
	Sound quality	Loud and high pitched
	Comparison of length of sound during respiration	Expiratory sounds are longer than inspiratory sounds
Tracheal	**Location of sound**	Trachea
	Sound quality	Loud and high pitched
	Comparison of length of sound during respiration	Inspiratory and expiratory sounds are equal
Bronchovesicular	**Location of sound**	Heard from the chest and between shoulder blades (scapulae)
	Sound quality	Medium pitch and intensity
	Comparison of length of sound during respiration	Inspiratory and expiratory sounds are equal
Vesicular	**Location of sound**	Both lungs in bronchioles and alveolar areas
	Sound quality	Low pitch and soft
	Comparison of sound during respiration	Fades away about one-third of the way through expiration

Abnormal (Adventitious) Sounds

Crackles *Also called rales*	Intermittent brief sounds with a nonmusical quality Described as fine or coarse Fine crackles: soft and high pitched; sound "explosive" Coarse crackles: louder and low pitched; sound "bubbly"
Rhonchi	Low-pitched sound that resembles snoring Can be caused by secretions or airway narrowing Usually disappears after coughing
Stridor	Sounds musical, similar to wheezing More prominent in inspiration Caused by upper airway obstruction Can be accompanied by use of accessory muscles
Wheezes	Continuous and musical High pitched Caused by airway narrowing

Data from Bickley L, Szilagyi P. The thorax and lungs. In: Bickley L, Szilagyi P. *Bates' Guide to Physical Examination and History Taking.* 10th ed. Philadelphia, PA: Lippincott Williams & Wilkins; 2009:283–321; Jones R. Respiratory system. In: Jones R, Rospond R, eds. *Patient Assessment in Pharmacy Practice.* Baltimore, MD: Lippincott Williams & Wilkins; 2003:186–212.

The Physical Exam

Auscultation of the lungs with a stethoscope is the best way to listen to lung sounds (Figure 8-3); however, it should be noted that in some instances lung sounds can be loud enough to be heard without a stethoscope. Therefore, even though a pharmacist may not regularly use a stethoscope in his or her normal practice, the pharmacist can listen for lung sounds while in the presence of the patient. Other presenting symptoms will help determine proper care for the patient presenting with abnormal lung sounds. For example, a patient with a history of asthma or COPD may experience wheezing periodically. After speaking with the physician, he or she may already have a plan on how to manage times of increased wheezing, and therefore can manage the problem without seeking help from the primary care provider. On the other hand, a person in which the symptom is new, or if the symptom continues or worsens despite treatment, should be referred to the primary care provider. It should be noted that, in some instances, lung obstruction can be so severe that very little air is able to flow through the lungs. In these situations, one may not hear abnormal lung sounds (Bickley, 2009). In these situations, the presence of accompanying symptoms, such as shortness of breath, coughing, or cyanosis, should dictate triage decisions.

How to Listen to the Lungs

1. Instruct the patient to sit upright with arms resting on his or her lap.
2. Ask the patient to inhale and exhale slowly and deeply through the mouth. Instruct the patient to stop if he or she begins to feel lightheaded or dizzy.
3. Stand behind the patient in a manner that will allow full view of the patient's back.
4. Place the diaphragm of the stethoscope on the patient's back at the #1 position (see **FIGURE 8-3**). While at this position, listen for breath sounds as the patient makes one full inhalation and one full exhalation.
5. After one full breath cycle, move the diaphragm to the opposite side of the back in the corresponding #1 position. Listen again for breath sounds. Continue this process down the back.

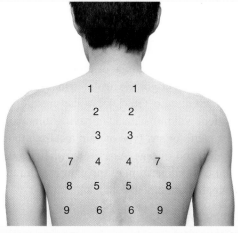

FIGURE 8-3 How to listen to the lungs.
© Kavee Vivii/Shutterstock, Inc.

Cough

Cough is a normal mechanism of the body designed to help keep the lungs and airways clear from a buildup of mucus, airway secretions, and foreign materials. An increase in frequency of cough or an increase in intensity of cough could signify an acute or chronic illness. A cough can be described as productive, which is when the cough results in the expulsion of mucus or airway secretions, or nonproductive, in which nothing is expelled with the cough. Nonproductive cough is also referred to as dry cough.

The Patient Interview

Questions in the patient interview should help differentiate between coughing that warrants medical treatment and coughing that can be treated with self-care practices. One should inquire as to whether the cough is productive or not. If the cough is productive, a follow-up question should be related to the quality and character of the material that is being expelled from the lungs as a result of the cough. If the cough is not productive, or is described as a dry cough, a follow-up question should be related to if the patient feels chest congestion. It is also important to ask questions related to the presence of other symptoms. Symptoms such as watery eyes, runny nose, and headache could suggest a viral infection, such as a common cold (Jones, 2003).

Hemoptysis:
Expelling blood as a result of coughing.

Asking about **hemoptysis**, or coughing up blood, is important. Reasons for coughing up blood can vary, and can be the result of bronchitis, pneumonia, or more serious conditions such as pulmonary embolism or cancer. For this reason, if the patient states that he or she is coughing up blood, it is important to try to quantify the amount by asking further questions, and to refer the patient for immediate medical attention (Bickley, 2009).

The Physical Exam

Coughing is a symptom that can be fully assessed by the pharmacist without the use of physical exam techniques. If coughing accompanies other symptoms, such as wheezing, shortness of breath, or pain, then a physical exam related to those particular complaints may be warranted.

Pain and the Pulmonary System

The origins of pain related to the pulmonary system may vary. Pain can be the result of excessive coughing, pneumonia, or pulmonary embolism. Pain can also be musculoskeletal or cardiac in origin. Gastrointestinal problems, such as heartburn and gastroesophageal reflux disease (GERD), can also present with pain in the chest area (Karnath, 2004). A patient will not state, "I'm having lung pain"; rather, they will report, "I am having chest pain" for any type of pain localized in the area of the body that includes the lungs, heart, and ribcage. As a result, when a patient presents with chest pain, it is important to try to determine if the pain is pulmonary, cardiac, musculoskeletal, or gastrointestinal in origin.

The Patient Interview

The patient interview should focus first and foremost on identifying if the pain is cardiac in origin. Cardiac pain could be suggestive of myocardial infarction, or heart attack, which warrants immediate emergency care.

Once it has been determined that the patient is most likely not experiencing cardiac pain, and is experiencing symptoms suggestive of pulmonary-related pain, the patient interview should be geared toward determining if the pain warrants medical attention or can be managed by self-care practices. If the patient reports that she or he is currently suffering from or has recently recovered from cough due to upper respiratory tract infection or cold in which they experienced a lot of coughing, it is possible that the pain being experienced is due to sore muscles engaged in the coughing mechanism. When one coughs, many muscles in the abdomen, chest, and back are engaged. Repeated coughing as well as the force exerted when coughing can cause pain. Asking the patient about the presence of associated symptoms, such as dyspnea, fever, chills or sweats, tachycardia, and cough, may help determine the best plan for seeking care.

Asking the patient about the location, character, and severity of the pain is helpful, too. Pain related to pneumonia can be described as a sharp pain that gets worse with coughing or when taking a deep breath (Lee, 2012). A sudden onset of sharp pain on one side of the chest in the absence of symptoms such as fever or other symptoms of a cold, but accompanied by shortness of breath, could be suggestive of **pneumothorax**, a condition that should also be treated immediately (Lee, 2012; Karnath, 2004). A quick assessment of the severity of pain can be performed by asking the patient to rate the pain on a scale of 1–10.

Pneumothorax: A condition in which air or gas accumulates in the pleural space in the lung cavity.

The Physical Exam

The patient interview can provide enough valuable information to help determine the origin, severity, and proper care for the patient's pain; however, observation of the patient experiencing pain related to the pulmonary system will also provide valuable information. For example, a patient with pulmonary-related pain may lean toward one particular side as a way to help relieve or prevent further pain on the affected side. In addition, observe if the patient is experiencing other pulmonary-related symptoms, such as cyanosis, wheezing, coughing, or changes in respiratory rate.

Asthma

Asthma is a chronic lung condition characterized by intermittent or persistent episodes of airway constriction. Pulmonary symptoms related to asthma include coughing, wheezing, and shortness of breath. Occurrences of asthma symptoms or worsening of persistent symptoms are referred to as asthma exacerbations or "asthma attacks." Depending on the severity, asthma exacerbations can be treated at home, in an urgent care center, at a physician's office, or in the emergency room. Severe asthma episodes that are unresponsive to treatment may require hospitalization for management (National Asthma Education and Prevention Program, 2007).

The Patient Interview

The patient interview for asthma will vary depending on whether the pharmacist is trying to assess an asthma exacerbation or the status of the chronic illness. The core questions are valuable in helping to assess an asthma exacerbation. Because asthma exacerbations can be triggered by exposure to certain allergens or irritants, asking the patient if the symptoms started after exposure to an allergen or irritant can provide valuable information. Many patients with asthma have been instructed to begin rescue therapy with a *beta$_2$*

Case #1

HP is a 28-year-old woman who has been referred to the pharmacotherapy clinic for asthma education. Before you begin the education session, you notice that she is breathing at a pace that is faster than normal. You also can hear that she is wheezing.

Questions

1. What additional measures could you take to assess the patient for symptoms of breathing difficulty?
2. What additional questions can you ask the patient to further assess this issue?

agonist inhaler, such as albuterol, at the start of symptoms (National Asthma Education and Prevention Program, 2007). The pharmacist should ask the patient if he or she began using the rescue inhaler at the start of symptoms and if the inhaler provided any relief of the symptoms.

The patient interview related to chronic asthma control really focuses on assessing the level of impairment and risk due to asthma. Questions related to the presence of symptoms during the day and night, and use of the rescue inhaler should be included in the interview. Also, the pharmacist should ask questions related to interference or limitations in daily activities and exercise due to asthma. To determine risk, the pharmacist should inquire about the number of exacerbations experienced and the number of exacerbations that required oral corticosteroids for treatment (National Asthma Education and Prevention Program, 2007).

The Physical Exam

During an asthma exacerbation, the main concern is related to the patient's ability to breathe and perfuse oxygen through the body. As such, the same physical exam techniques used to assess respiration are used for an asthma exacerbation. Observing the patient for the presence of cyanosis, tripod stance, agitation, and confusion is key. Listening for the presence of wheezing with or without the use of a stethoscope can also be performed, keeping in mind that not all patients with asthma will experience wheezing and that the presence or absence of wheezing does not correlate to the severity of exacerbation. Observing the patient's ability to speak in full sentences is also an important assessment during an asthma exacerbation.

Clinical Presentation of Drug-Induced Processes

A number of medications have been found to cause pulmonary disorders. In most cases, the clinical presentation of these disorders is very similar to the clinical presentation of other pulmonary conditions; as a result, the idea that the disorder may be drug-related is either overlooked or ranked lower on the list of potential causes. When a patient presents with pulmonary symptoms that are atypical for the patient's age, if the patient doesn't fit the risk factors for the condition, or if the patient does not seem to respond to typical therapy for the condition, begin to investigate the patient's medication list for possible drug-induced causes of the condition.

Opioid-Induced Respiratory Depression

Opioids have a long history of being used for pain management following surgery and for the management of various disease states. However, one of the major side effects of using opioids is respiratory depression. Management of this concern involves regular monitoring of the patient's respiratory status and assuring that the opioid dose administered to the patient is the lowest, most effective dose to manage that patient's pain (Hartkopf Smith, 2007). For cases of respiratory depression that warrant immediate reversal, administration of naloxone is suggested (Dahan, 2007, 2010). Risk factors for respiratory depression due to opioid use are shown in **Table 8-3**.

Table 8-3 Risk Factors for Opioid-Induced Respiratory Depression

Age > 65	Renal dysfunction
Liver disease	Sleep apnea
Pulmonary disease	Obesity
Heart disease	Smoker
Increased sedation	Opioid naïve
Concurrent use of CNS depressants	

Data from Hartkopf Smith L. Opioid safety: is your patient at risk for respiratory depression? *Clin J Oncol Nurs.* 2007;11(2):293–296.

ACE Inhibitor–Induced Cough

Angiotensin-converting enzyme (ACE) inhibitors have an established history in causing cough (Overlack, 1996). ACE inhibitor–induced cough is described as a chronic, dry, nonproductive cough. Patients experiencing this phenomenon will often describe the cough as being precipitated by a tickling sensation in the throat (Overlack, 1996). The onset of cough varies from hours after the initial dose to months into treatment. Per ACCP clinical practice guidelines (2006), discontinuation of the medication will lead to resolution of the problem in usually 1 to 4 weeks, but can take as long as 3 months to resolve. ACE inhibitor–induced cough should be considered in patients who present with a dry cough and are currently being treated with medication in this drug class. The suspicion of ACE inhibitor–induced cough should be high in circumstances when the patient does not have a diagnosis of lung disease that can cause cough, is afebrile, and does not present with other symptoms that would be suggestive of other illnesses.

Pulmonary Disorders Related to Illicit Drug Use

Pharmacists should also be aware that some illicit drugs can cause pulmonary complications. Illicit drug use should be on the list of possible causes of pulmonary diseases, especially if an underlying cause cannot be identified or if the patient is presenting with a pulmonary condition that typically does not occur in the patient's age range or the patient does not have risk factors that typically are seen with the illness.

Pulmonary complications of illicit drug use are not limited to those drugs administered by inhalation. Intravenous administration of illicit drugs can cause pulmonary complications as well. Talcosis, an interstitial lung disease caused by the inhalation of talcum powder, can develop in persons who use illicit drugs in which talcum powder has been added to the drug as an additive to increase the weight of the product. Talcosis can also occur when people crush tablets meant for oral consumption and snort or use them intravenously. Symptoms can range from cough and shortness of breath to pulmonary hypertension or chronic respiratory failure (Scheel, 2012; Marchiori, 2010). Pulmonary embolism due to foreign bodies can occur if a portion of the talc or other ingredient used during inhalation or intravenous administration lodges in the lung (Weiner, 2011). Inhaling crack can cause a number of lung conditions, including pulmonary edema, "crack lung," interstitial pneumonitis, and bronchiolitis obliterans with organizing pneumonia. Crack lung is a condition characterized by hypoxemia, dyspnea, fever, hemoptysis, and respiratory failure (Devlin, 2008; Haim, 1995; Forrester, 1990).

Cultural Considerations for the Pulmonary Assessment

Cultural Approaches to Assessing Cyanosis

A hallmark sign of cyanosis in a patient is the bluish color typically observed by viewing areas on the skin and around the mucus membranes. However, depending on the patient's skin tone, cyanotic areas of the skin may not look blue to the person observing the patient. The characteristic blue hue can be seen in patients with white or lighter toned skin; however, cyanotic skin in a patient with darker skin tones may appear grayish or white (Beckmann, 2008; Sommers, 2011). One should look for the presence of a grayish or greenish hue on the earlobes, lips, or nail beds as a sign of cyanosis in patients with lighter skin tones (Beckmann, 2008; Sommers, 2011) (**FIGURE 8-4**). The presence of bluish, grayish, or pale skin on the conjunctiva, lips, tongue, palms, or soles of the feet can signify cyanosis in patients with darker skin tones (Beckman, 2008).

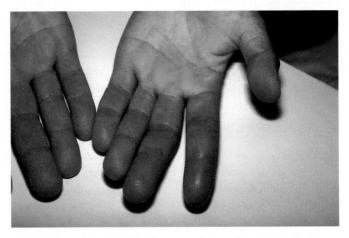

FIGURE 8-4 Alternate sites to assess for cyanosis. Observe the marked appearance of the bluish, purple hue on the pads of the fingers.
© ISM/Phototake, Inc.

Cultural Considerations Regarding Asthma Management

Understanding a patient's explanatory model for asthma can help to better assess a patient and provide culturally relevant care. Learning about the patient's beliefs regarding why they have asthma (**Table 8-4**), as well as how they believe it should be treated, is an important step in the assessment process. Therefore, asking a patient questions such as "Why do you think you have asthma?" "What does it mean when you have asthma?" or "What do you think caused this asthma episode or attack?" may help to gather more insight on the patient's belief about the condition.

Table 8-4 Reported Reasons Patients May Believe They Have Asthma

Environmental factors
Genetics
Stress
Inappropriate dressing in cold weather
Spiritual reasons (e.g., test of faith or punishment)

Data from George M, Birck K, Hufford D, Jemmott L, Weaver T. Beliefs about asthma and complementary and alternative medicine in low-income inner-city African-American adults. *J Gen Intern Med.* 2006;21:1317–1324.

Similar to other chronic diseases, asthma is a condition in which proper management involves not only medication use, but also self-management practices that the patient must employ. Therefore, it is important to review with the patient self-management practices used to manage asthma and to weigh whether the techniques they are currently using could help with asthma management or potentially cause harm to the patient. Complementary and alternative medicine (CAM) practices have been used by various cultural groups to manage asthma (Bearison, 2002; George, 2009; Cotton, 2011; Rivera, 2004). CAM methods include performing breathing exercises and relaxation techniques, prayer, use of vitamins and herbal products, and home remedies (**Table 8-5**).

Table 8-5 Reported CAM Methods Used to Help Manage Asthma

Camphor or mentholated chest rubs applied topically or ingested
Fluid intake (water, coffee, tea with lemon, honey, or alcohol)
Staying out of cold or wet weather
Inhaling steam
Chest percussion
Prayer
Relaxation
Getting fresh air

Data from George M, Birck K, Hufford D, Jemmott L, Weaver T. Beliefs about asthma and complementary and alternative medicine in low-income inner-city African-American adults. *J Gen Intern Med.* 2006;21:1317–1324; George M, Campbell J, Rand C. Self-management of acute asthma among low-income urban adults. *J Asthma.* 2009;46:618–624; Cotton S, Luberto C, Yi M, Tsevat J. Complementary and alternative medicine behaviors and beliefs in urban adolescents with asthma. *J Asthma.* 2011;48:531–538.

As a pharmacist, utilizing an explanatory model type question such as "What do you think is the best way to treat this condition?" can help gain insight on CAM use and the role the patient believes CAM plays in the management of asthma. In some instances, however, the patient may not share information about CAM techniques used; therefore, the pharmacist may introduce the idea by asking the patient if they use other methods to treat asthma other than prescription medication (Bearison, 2002; Cotton, 2011; Rivera, 2004). It would also be important to ask the patient if CAM is used along with prescribed asthma medications or instead of prescribed asthma medications (George, 2009). If the prescribed medications are used along with CAM, asking the patient whether he or she adjusts the medication dose can provide insight on whether there is overuse or underuse of the prescription medication, as well as if the patient's regimen is adequately controlling the asthma or causing harm (Bearison, 2002; George, 2006). In addition, asking the patient if the severity of the asthma symptoms plays a role in the choice of CAM or use of prescription medications can be useful (Bearison, 2002; George, 2009). When asking this question, it is important for the pharmacist to be able to understand how the patient defines severity of their asthma (George, 2009). Therefore, asking the patient questions such as "What would you consider to be an asthma attack that is bad (severe) versus one that is not so bad (mild)?" and "How would you treat a bad asthma attack compared to one that is not so bad?" can be helpful.

Summary

The pharmacist's role in assessing the pulmonary system includes performing a patient interview and a limited physical assessment. Interviewing the patient is a valuable way to gather information; however, observation of the patient is just as valuable because lung-related conditions can affect posture and the ability to speak in full sentences. Being aware of cultural beliefs and practices regarding asthma management and inquiring about them during the patient visit can lead to more culturally appropriate patient care.

Review Questions

1. You are on a plane to Florida for a pharmacy conference. You notice that your seatmate begins taking rapid but prolonged, deep breaths just as the plane ascends into the air. Is your seatmate most likely experiencing tachypnea or hyperventilation? What information supports your answer?

2. A 48-year-old woman goes to the pharmacy to pick up a prescription medication. While there, she explains to the pharmacist that she has been experiencing chest pain for 2 days. After a thorough interview, the pharmacist determined that her chest pain warrants further investigation, and therefore suggests that she go to the urgent care center. At the urgent care center the doctors were able to determine that her chest pain was not cardiac in nature, but of pulmonary origin. What could have been the possible signs or symptoms the patient expressed to warrant the pharmacist's suggestion?

References

Bearison D, Minian N, Granowetter L. Medical management of asthma and folk medicine in a Hispanic community. *J Pediatr Psychol*. 2002;27:385–392.

Bickley L, Szilagyi P. Beginning the physical examination: general survey, vital signs, and pain. In: Bickley L, Szilagyi P, eds. *Bates' Guide to Physical Examination and History Taking*. 10th ed. Philadelphia, PA: Lippincott Williams & Wilkins; 2009:101–134.

Bickley L, Szilagyi P. The thorax and lungs. In: Bickley L, Szilagyi P, eds. *Bates' Guide to Physical Examination and History Taking*. 10th ed. Philadelphia, PA: Lippincott Williams & Wilkins; 2009:283–321.

Bauldoff G. When breathing is a burden: how to help patients with COPD. *American Nurse Today*. 2012;7(8):17–23.

Cotton S, Luberto C, Yi M, Tsevat J. Complementary and alternative medicine behaviors and beliefs in urban adolescents with asthma. *J Asthma*. 2011;48:531–538.

Dahan A, Aarts L, Smith T. Incidence, reversal, and prevention of opioid-induced respiratory depression. *Anesthesiology*. 2010;112(1):226–238.

Dahan A. Respiratory depression with opioids. *J Pain Palliat Care Pharmacother*. 2007;21:63–66.

Devlin R, Henry J. Clinical review: Major consequences of illicit drug consumption. *Crit Care*. 2008;12(1):202. doi: 10.1186/cc6166. Epub 2008 Jan 8.

Dicpinigaitis PV. Angiotensin-converting enzyme inhibitor-induced cough: ACCP evidence-based clinical practice guidelines. *CHEST*. 2006;129(1 Suppl):169S–173S.

Forrester JM, Steele AW, Waldron JA, Parsons PE. Crack lung: an acute pulmonary syndrome with a spectrum of clinical and histopathologic findings. *Am Rev Respir Dis*. 1990;142(2):462–467.

George M, Birck K, Hufford D, Jemmott L, Weaver T. Beliefs about asthma and complementary and alternative medicine in low-income inner-city African-American adults. *J Gen Intern Med*. 2006;21:1317–1324.

George M, Campbell, J, Rand C. Self-management of acute asthma among low-income urban adults. *J Asthma*. 2009;46:618–624.

Haim DY, Lippmann ML, Goldberg SK, Walkenstein MD. The pulmonary complications of crack cocaine. A comprehensive review. *Chest*. 1995;107(1):233–240.

Hartkopf Smith L. Opioid safety: Is your patient at risk for respiratory depression? *Clin J Oncol Nurs*. 2007;11(2):293–296.

Jones, R. General assessment and vital signs. In: Jones R, Rospond R, eds. *Patient Assessment in Pharmacy Practice*. Baltimore, MD: Lippincott Williams & Wilkins; 2003:43–61.

Jones R. Respiratory system. In: Jones R, Rospond R, eds. *Patient Assessment in Pharmacy Practice*. Baltimore, MD: Lippincott Williams & Wilkins; 2003:186–212.

Karnath B, Holden M, Hussain N. Chest pain: differentiating cardiac from noncardiac causes. *Hospital Physician*. 2004:40(4):24–27.

Lee TH. Chest discomfort. In: Fauci AS, Kasper DL, Jameson JL, Longo DL, Hauser SL, eds. *Harrison's Principles of Internal Medicine*. 18th ed. New York: McGraw-Hill; 2012. Available at: http://www.accesspharmacy.com/content.aspx?aID=9094636. Accessed February 28, 2013.

Marchiori E, Lourenco S, Gasparetto T, Zanetti G, Mano C, Nobre L. Pulmonary talcosis: imaging findings. *Lung*. 2010;188(2):165–171. Epub 2010 Feb 13.

National Asthma Education and Prevention Program, Third Expert Panel on the Diagnosis and Management of Asthma. *Expert Panel Report 3: Guidelines for the Diagnosis and Management of Asthma*. Bethesda, MD: National Heart, Lung, and Blood Institute; 2007.

Overlack A. ACE inhibitor-induced cough and bronchospasm. Incidence, mechanisms and management. *Drug Safety*. 1996;15(1):72–78.

Rivera J, Hughes H, Stuart A. Herbals and asthma: usage patterns among a border population. *Ann Pharmacother*. 2004;38:220–225.

Scheel A, Krause D, Haars H, Schmitz I, Junker K. Talcum induced pneumoconiosis following inhalation of adulterated marijuana, a case report. *Diagn Pathol*. 2012;7:26. doi: 10.1186/1746-1596-7-26.

Sociocultural Influences. In: Beckmann Murray R, Proctor Zentner J, and Yakimo R. *Health Promotion Strategies Through the Lifespan*. 8th ed. Prentice Hall: New Jersey; 2008:139 accessed at http://wps.prenhall.com/wps/media/objects/6356/6509531/tools/table5-12.pdf.

Sommers M. Color awareness: a must for patient assessment. *Am Nurs Today*. 2011;6(1). Available at: http://www.medscape.com/viewarticle/741045. Accessed March 1, 2013.

Weiner J, Chandak TR, Fein A. A Case of fatal pulmonary and systemic talc embolism [Abstract]. Great Cases: Clinical, Radiologic and Pathologic Correlations by master physicians. In: Proceedings of the American Thoracic Society International Conference; May 13–18, 2011; Denver, Colorado. Abstract 83.

Chapter 9

Neurologic Assessment
Yolanda M. Hardy, PharmD

LEARNING OBJECTIVES

At the completion of this chapter, the reader should be able to:

1. Determine appropriate questions to ask patients when performing a focused nervous system patient interview.
2. Explain the clinical presentation of common symptoms and diseases related to the nervous system.
3. Explain how to correctly perform the physical assessment techniques related to the nervous system.
4. List medications that can cause adverse effects or medical conditions affecting the nervous system.
5. Explain the clinical presentation of drug-induced disease processes.
6. Triage patients based on clinical presentation of problems related to the nervous system.
7. Explain cultural considerations, particularly related to the elderly population in regard to falls.

KEY TERMS

Disequilibrium

Lightheadedness

Presyncope

Vertigo

Introduction

The nervous system, which consists of the brain, spinal cord, and nerves, plays a role in all functions of the body. Injury or disease affecting any part of the nervous system can manifest itself in different ways, ranging from producing symptoms of illness to loss of functionality of body parts or systems. As a result, there is a vast array of conditions that can have their origins in the nervous system. This chapter will discuss general conditions of the nervous system that the pharmacist may commonly experience in daily practice.

© ontishock/Shutterstock, Inc.

Depending on the clinical presentation, interviewing the patient by asking questions related to onset, location, duration, character, aggravating factors, relieving factors, timing, and severity of symptoms may prove beneficial. Additional questions related to how the condition is affecting the patient's lifestyle and ability to perform daily tasks may be important based on the condition.

Physical assessment by the pharmacist will vary based on the patient's clinical presentation. In some cases a patient interview will provide enough information; in other instances a physical assessment can be performed. Depending on the cause of the condition or the symptoms the patient presents with, a referral to the primary care provider may be warranted.

Clinical Presentation of Symptoms and Disease Processes Related to the Nervous System

Dizziness

Vertigo:
A sensation in which one perceives that his or her surroundings are moving or spinning.

Disequilibrium:
A sensation of feeling off-balance.

Presyncope:
A sensation in which one feels as if he or she will faint.

Lightheadedness:
A sensation of feeling unsteady on one's feet. Sometimes accompanied by the sensation of feeling as if one is about to faint.

The term *dizzy* should be viewed as a general term patients use to describe one of many sensations. According to Post (2010), dizziness can be classified as **vertigo, disequilibrium, presyncope,** or **lightheadedness** (**Table 9-1**). Vertigo is characterized as having a sensation that the environment is moving or spinning (Walker, 2012; Post, 2010). Disequilibrium is described as feeling "off-balance." Presyncope is the sensation of feeling like one is going to faint or pass out. Descriptions for lightheadedness are not as clear. The patient may describe feeling "out of sorts" or as if they are floating. A patient may experience one type of dizziness or a combination of multiple types at the same time.

Table 9-1 Selected Causes of Dizziness

Disequilibrium	
Parkinson's disease	Alterations in gait can cause imbalance, which can lead to falls.
Peripheral neuropathy	Decreased sensation in feet can alter perceptions when walking, which can lead to imbalance and falls.
Lightheadedness	
Hyperventilation syndrome	Sensation that occurs as a result of experiencing hyperventilation, which can be due to anxiety or emotional conditions or situations.
Presyncope	
Orthostatic hypotension	A drop in blood pressure that can be a result of decreased blood flow to the brain or using medications that can lower blood pressure. It is noted by a 20 mm Hg decrease in systolic blood pressure or a 10 mm Hg decrease in diastolic blood pressure or an increase in pulse by 30 beats per minute.
Vertigo	
Benign paroxysmal positional vertigo	Causes a false sensation of motion upon positional changes of the head.
Meniere's disease	Results from a disorder that is characterized by fluid buildup in the inner ear.

Data from Post R, Dickerson L. Dizziness: a diagnostic approach. *Am Fam Physician*. 2010;82(4):361–368.

Case #1

While working in the community pharmacy, you notice that JR, a 68-year-old man and long-time client of the pharmacy, stands up from his chair in the waiting area and stumbles upon his approach to the pharmacy counter. JR then holds onto the pharmacy counter for balance, and begins to shake his head. Concerned, you ask JR if he is ok. JR tells you that he is fine, he just felt a little "woozy." He states that he has been experiencing "dizzy spells" over the past week whenever he stands up.

Question

1. What questions would you like to ask JR in order to gather more information about his dizzy spells?

The Patient Interview

The first step during the patient interview is to try to determine exactly what the patient is experiencing when he or she complains of dizziness (Post, 2010; Kerber, 2011). Asking the patient to describe what he or she is feeling will provide the pharmacist with an idea of the type of dizziness that the person is dealing with. Pharmacists should also inquire about recent head trauma and recent automobile accidents that may have caused whiplash (Tameem, 2013). The pharmacist should also inquire about falls, both for the purpose of determining if the fall was the cause of the dizziness (i.e., as a result of head injury due to the fall) or if the fall was as a result of being dizzy (Benson, 2012).

At some point, every person will experience an episode of dizziness. However, new onset dizziness, dizziness that is recurrent or continuous, dizziness that occurs after recent head injury, or reports of additional symptoms such as nausea, shortness of breath, or weakness in the extremities all warrant further follow-up with the patient's primary care provider as these symptoms suggest that the dizziness is a sign of a more serious condition.

The Physical Exam

The physical exam for dizziness may include an exam of the cardiovascular system and the neurologic system. The exam may involve assessing for orthostatic hypotension or cardiac abnormalities and performing various neurological tests to check for nystagmus or alterations in coordination or balance (Goebel, 2001; Kerber, 2011). Because of this, it is best for this type of examination to be reserved for the patient's primary care provider or neurologist.

Fall Risk

Issues with gait or balance can place a patient at risk of falling. Elderly patients are at an increased risk of falling and also are at higher risk of complications if they do suffer a fall (Fuller, 2000; CDC, 2013). Assessing patients, especially the elderly, for the risk of falling is one way to possibly prevent a fall from occurring. **Table 9-2** describes a number of risk factors that have been identified for falls.

The Patient Interview

The patient interview provides an opportunity for the pharmacist to screen a patient for fall risk. The interview should include questioning about the use of wheelchairs, canes, and walkers, both in the home and outside of the home. The pharmacist should also

Table 9-2 Risk Factors for Falls

Patient-Related Factors	Lifestyle Factors
Acute illness	Housebound
Age (especially ≥ 75 years)	Living alone
Chronic medical conditions, especially neuromuscular conditions	Use of canes or walkers
Cognitive impairment	
History of falls	
Medication use	
Neurologic changes	
Vision impairment	
White race	

Data from Fuller G. Falls in the elderly. *Am Fam Physician*. 2000;61(7):2159–2168; Studenski S, Wolter L. Instability and falls. In: Duthie EH Jr, Katz PR, eds. *Practice of Geriatrics*. 3rd ed. Philadelphia, PA: Saunders; 1998:199–206; Tinetti ME, Doucette J, Claus E, Marottoli R. Risk factors for serious injury during falls by older persons in the community. *J Am Geriatr Soc*. 1995;43:1214–1221.

ask whether the patient has experienced any falls in the past or episodes of tripping on things. A patient may consider falling only those occasions when he or she actually hit the ground, and therefore may not report episodes where he or she was able to catch him- or herself before falling to the ground. Therefore, it is important to inquire about falls that included falling to the ground and falls that did not include falling to the ground. The patient interview also should include questions about the use of area rugs or other items in the home that may increase the patient's risk of falling. Finally, the patient interview should also include questions about whether the patient has a fear of falling. A checklist, such as the one available from the National Center for Injury Prevention and Control (**Table 9-3**) is a helpful tool to use when interviewing a patient about falls.

Table 9-3 Home Fall Risk Assessment

Location	Questions to Ask	Suggestions for the Patient
Floors	When you walk through a room, do you have to walk around furniture?	Ask someone to move the furniture so your path is clear.
	Do you have throw rugs on the floor?	Remove the rugs or use double-sided tape or a nonslip backing so the rugs won't slip.
	Are there papers, books, towels, shoes, magazines, boxes, blankets, or other objects on the floor?	Pick up things that are on the floor. Always keep objects off the floor.
	Do you have to walk over or around wires or cords (like lamp, telephone, or extension cords)?	Coil or tape cords and wires next to the wall so you can't trip over them. If needed, have an electrician put in another outlet.

Table 9-3 Home Fall Risk Assessment *(continued)*

Location	Questions to Ask	Suggestions for the Patient
Kitchen	Are the things you use often on high shelves?	Move items in your cabinets. Keep things you use often on the lower shelves (about waist level).
	Is your step stool unsteady?	If you must use a step stool, get one with a bar to hold onto. Never use a chair as a step stool.
Bedrooms	Is the light near the bed hard to reach?	Place a lamp close to the bed where it is easy to reach.
	Is the path from your bed to the bathroom dark?	Put in a nightlight so you can see where you are walking. Some nightlights go on by themselves after dark.
Bathrooms	Is the tub or shower floor slippery?	Put a nonslip rubber mat or self-stick strips on the floor of the tub or shower.
	Do you need some support when you get into and out of the tub or up from the toilet?	Have a carpenter put grab bars inside the tub and next to the toilet.
Stairs and steps	Are there papers, shoes, books, or other objects on the stairs?	Pick up things on the stairs. Always keep objects off stairs.
	Are some steps broken or uneven?	Fix loose or uneven steps.
	Are you missing a light over the stairway?	Have an electrician put in an overhead light at the top and bottom of the stairs.
	Do you have only one light switch for your stairs (only at the top or at the bottom of the stairs)?	Have an electrician put in a light switch at the top and bottom of the stairs. You can get light switches that glow.
	Has the stairway light bulb burned out?	Have a friend or family member change the light bulb.
	Is the carpet on the steps loose or torn?	Make sure the carpet is firmly attached to every step, or remove the carpet and attach nonslip rubber treads to the stairs.
	Are the handrails loose or broken? Is there a handrail on only one side of the stairs?	Fix loose handrails or put in new ones. Make sure handrails are on both sides of the stairs and are as long as the stairs.

Reproduced from Centers for Disease Control, National Center for Injury Prevention and Control. Check for Safety: a home fall prevention checklist for older adults. Available at: http://www.cdc.gov/ncipc/pub-res/toolkit/checklistforsafety.htm. Accessed March 3, 2013.

The Physical Exam

A quick assessment that can be performed by the pharmacist is the Timed Up and Go (TUG) test by Podsiadlo and Richardson (1991). This test enables the clinician to assess the patient's gait, stability, balance, stride length, and sway. For this test, the pharmacist

Patient: _____ Date: _____ Time: _____ AM/PM

The Timed Up and Go (TUG) Test

Purpose: To assess mobility
Equipment: A stopwatch
Directions: Patients wear their regular footwear and can use a walking aid if needed. Begin by having the patient sit back in a standard arm chair and identify a line 3 meters or 10 feet away on the floor.

Instructions to the patient:

When I say "**Go**," I want you to:
1) Stand up from the chair
2) Walk to the line on the floor at your normal pace
3) Turn
4) Walk back to the chair at your normal pace
5) Sit down again

On the word "**Go**" begin timing.
Stop timing after patient has sat back down and record.

Time: _____ seconds

An older adult who takes ≥12 seconds to complete the TUG is at high risk for falling.

Observe the patient's postural stability, gait, stride length, and sway.

Circle all that apply: ☐ Slow tentative pace ☐ Loss of balance ☐ Short strides ☐ Little or no arm swing ☐ Steadying self on walls ☐ Shuffling ☐ En bloc turning ☐ Not using assistive device properly
Notes:

For relevant articles, go to: **www.cdc.gov/injury/STEADI**

FIGURE 9-1 Timed Up and Go test.

Reproduced from Centers for Disease Control. STEADI (Stopping elderly accidents, deaths and injuries) tool kit for health care providers. Available at: http://www.cdc.gov/homeandrecreationalsafety/Falls/steadi/index.html. Accessed May 16, 2014.

will determine how long it takes for a patient to get up from a seated position, walk 10 feet, turn around, walk back to the starting point, and return to a seated position (**FIGURE 9-1**). A person is considered at high risk for falling if it takes 12 or more seconds to complete the test. In addition to observing the length of time, the pharmacist should observe the patient's gait, posture, balance, and walking pattern. Mathias, Nayak, and Isaacs's (1986) Get Up and Go test is similar to the TUG, with the difference being that the time it takes to complete the task is not measured. Rather, a score is determined based on how the patient performed compared to normal performance (**FIGURE 9-2**). Because the patients most likely to be asked to perform these assessments are doing so because of their risk of fall, it is suggested that when the patient performs the test the pharmacist be close by

Get-up and Go Test

Instructions:
Ask the patient to perform the following series of maneuvers: 1) Sit comfortably in a straight-backed chair. 2) Rise from the chair. 3) Stand still momentarily. 4) Walk a short distance (approximately 3 meters). 5) Turn around. 6) Walk back to the chair. 7) Turn around. 8) Sit down in the chair.
Scoring:

Observe the patient's movements for any deviation from a confident, normal performance. Use the following scale:
 	
   1 = Normal
   2 = Very slightly abnormal
   3 = Mildly abnormal
   4 = Moderately abnormal
   5 = Severely abnormal
 	
"Normal" indicates that the patient gave no evidence of being at risk of falling during the test or at any other time. "Severely abnormal" indicates that the patient appeared at risk of falling during the test. Intermediate grades reflect the presence of any of the following as indicators of the possibility of falling: undue slowness, hesitancy, abnormal movements of the trunk or upper limbs, staggering, stumbling.
 	
A patient with a score of 3 or more on the Get-up and Go Test is at risk of falling.

FIGURE 9-2 Get Up and Go test.

Reproduced from Mathias S, Nayak USL, Isaacs B. Balance in elderly patients: the "get-up and go" test. *Arch Phys Med Rehabil.* 1986;67:387–389.

to assist the patient if he or she appears as if he or she may fall. Findings of these tests should be reported to the patient's healthcare provider.

Clinical Presentation of Drug-Induced Processes

Drug-Induced Dizziness and Falls

Multiple medications have been implicated in causing dizziness and falls (**Table 9-4**). Many of the medications that can cause dizziness can ultimately lead to falls in some patients. The patient interview provides a great opportunity for the pharmacist to review the patient's medication list and identify those medications that can cause dizziness or may increase the risk of falling. In the event that these medications must be prescribed, and there are no other alternatives with a safer profile, educating the patient on measures that could be taken to prevent falls is important (Cranwell-Bruce, 2008; Fuller, 2000).

Case #1 *(continued)*

After further questioning, JR tells you that he has made sure to remove things that would increase his chance of falling at home because his wife took a bad fall a year ago. Upon reading his medication profile, you notice that a week ago he was given a new prescription for the antihypertensive medication amlodipine and his hydrochlorothiazide dose was also increased.

Question

2. What is the most likely cause of JR's dizzy spells?

Table 9-4 Medications That May Increase the Risk of Falling

Medications for Mental Health Conditions	Medications for Cardiovascular Conditions	Other Agents
Benzodiazepines Tricyclic antidepressants Phenothiazines (e.g., thorazine, thioridazine, and prochlorperazine) Butyrophenones (e.g., haloperidol and droperidol)	Antihypertensives Cardiac agents	Anticholinergic agents Corticosteroids Eye drops Hypoglycemic agents Nonsteroidal anti-inflammatory agents

Data from Fuller G. Falls in the elderly. *Am Fam Physician*. 2000;61(7):2159–2168.

Cultural Considerations with the Nervous System

If the elderly population is viewed as a culture, one can postulate that this culture is at risk for falls. In addition to risk of falling, the fear of falling is also present in some elderly patients. The perceived risk of falling also varies within the elderly population (Delbaere, 2010; Deshpande, 2009; Legters, 2002; Howland, 1993). Therefore, during the patient interview, the pharmacist should inquire not only about fall risk, but also about fear of falling. Asking the patient if they ever think about, fear, or worry about falling would be a good way to initiate the conversation (Legters, 2002).

As pharmacists, it is important for us to realize that having a fear of falling can significantly affect an elderly person's lifestyle (Delbaere, 2004; Yardley, 2012). Pharmacists should be aware that this may impact how other disease states are managed. For example, it is common to recommend exercise as part of the treatment of many diseases, such as hypertension and diabetes. If a patient has a fear of falling that has limited their level of comfort with physical activity, then recommending general exercise should be done while considering the patient's fear of falling.

Summary

Dizziness and falls are two conditions related to the nervous system that are due to various causes, including medication use. Interviewing a patient who complains of dizziness and reviewing medication records can help determine if the cause is drug related. Assessing a patient's risk for falling and fear of falling, and investigating their use of medications that have been known to increase the risk for falls are two valuable practices that can be done to help lower the risk for falling.

Review Questions

1. A patient presents to the pharmacy complaining of dizziness. Which questions would you ask to gather more information about her complaint?
2. You are a home infusion pharmacist who is scheduled to visit SW, a 70-year-old woman who is being treated for cellulitis. SW walks with a cane in public and has a walker to use at home. When you arrive at her home, you notice that the

concrete stairs leading to her door are crumbling. When you ring the doorbell, it takes a while for SW to answer. When she does, you notice that she is not using her walker. Upon entering SW's home, you notice that her living area is small, and the floors are covered with rugs. She has large pieces of furniture in the living area, which take up most of the free space in the room. In addition to the antibiotics for the cellulitis, SW is also taking an antihypertensive for her blood pressure, an analgesic for arthritis, and a benzodiazepine for sleep. Based on this information, how would you assess SW's risk for fall? Why?

References

Benson B, Busino R, Sidor M, Baredes S. Posttraumatic vertigo. Medscape. Available at: http://emedicine.medscape.com/article/884361-overview. Updated March 1, 2012. Accessed August 18, 2014.

Centers for Disease Control and Prevention. Falls among older adults: an overview. Home and Recreational Safety. Available at: http://www.cdc.gov/homeandrecreationalsafety/falls/adultfalls.html. Updated 2013. Accessed August 16, 2014.

Centers for Disease Control. STEADI (Stopping elderly accidents, deaths and injuries) tool kit for health care providers. Available at: http://www.cdc.gov/homeandrecreationalsafety/Falls/steadi/index.html. Accessed May 16, 2014.

Centers for Disease Control and Prevention. The timed up and go (TUG) test. Available at: http://www.cdc.gov/homeandrecreationalsafety/pdf/steadi/timed_up_and_go_test.pdf. Accessed April 17, 2014.

Centers for Disease Control, National Center for Injury Prevention and Control. Check for safety: a home fall prevention checklist for older adults. Available at: http://www.cdc.gov/ncipc/pub-res/toolkit/checklistforsafety.htm. Accessed March 3, 2013.

Cranwell-Bruce L. The connection between patient falls and medication. *Medsurg Nursing.* 2008;17(3):189–191.

Delbaere K, Close J, Brodaty H, Sachdev P, Lord S. Determinants of disparities between perceived and physiological risk of falling among elderly people: cohort study. *BMJ.* 2010;341:c4165.

Delbaere K, Crombez G, Vanderstraeten G, Willems T, Cambier D. Fear-related avoidance of activities, falls and physical frailty. A prospective community-based cohort study. *Age Ageing* 2004;33:368–373.

Deshpande N, Metter E, Lauretani F, Bandinelli S, Ferruchi L. Interpreting fear of falling in the elderly: what do we need to consider? *J Geriatr Phys Ther.* 2009;32(3):91–96.

Fuller G. Falls in the elderly. *Am Fam Physician.* 2000;61(7):2159–2168.

Goebel J. The ten-minute examination of the dizzy patient. *Semin Neurol.* 2001;21(4):391–398.

Howland J, Peterson EW, Levin WC, Fried L, Pordon D, Bak S. Fear of falling among the community-dwelling elderly. *J Aging Health.* 1993;5:229–243.

Kerber KA, Baloh RW. The evaluation of a patient with dizziness. *Neurol Clin Pract.* 2011;1(1):24–33.

Legters K. Fear of falling. *Phys Ther.* 2002;82:264–272.

Mathias S, Nayak USL, Isaacs B. Balance in elderly patients: the "get-up and go" test. *Arch Phys Med Rehabil.* 1986;67:387–389.

National Institutes of Health Senior Health. Falls and older adults. Available at: http://nihseniorhealth.gov/falls/causesandriskfactors/01.html. Updated January 2013. Accessed August 16, 2014.

Podsiadlo D, Richardson S. The timed "Up & Go": a test of basic functional mobility for frail elderly persons. *J Am Geriatr Soc.* 1991;39:142–148.

Post R, Dickerson L. Dizziness: a diagnostic approach. *Am Fam Physician.* 2010;82(4):361–368.

Tameem A, Kapur S, Mutagi H. Whiplash injury. *Contin Educ Anaesth Crit Care Pain.* 2013:1–4. doi: 10.1093/bjaceaccp/mkt052.

Walker MF, Daroff RB. Dizziness and vertigo. In: Fauci AS, Kasper DL, Jameson JL, Longo DL, Hauser SL, eds. *Harrison's Principles of Internal Medicine.* 18th ed. New York: McGraw-Hill; 2012. Available at: http://www.accesspharmacy.com/content.aspx?aID=9096086. Accessed March 3, 2013.

Yardley L, Smith H. A prospective study of the relationship between feared consequences of falling and avoidance of activity in community-living older people. *Gerontologist.* 2002;42:17–23.

Chapter 10

Peripheral Vascular Assessment
Yolanda M. Hardy, PharmD

LEARNING OBJECTIVES

At the completion of this chapter, the reader should be able to:

1. Determine appropriate questions to ask patients when performing a focused peripheral vascular system interview.
2. Explain the clinical presentation of common symptoms and diseases related to the peripheral vascular system.
3. Explain how to correctly perform the physical assessment techniques related to the peripheral vascular system.
4. List medications that can cause adverse effects or medical conditions affecting the peripheral vascular system.
5. Explain the clinical presentation of drug-induced disease processes.
6. Triage patients based on clinical presentation of problems related to the peripheral vascular system.
7. Discuss health disparities related to amputations resulting from peripheral vascular conditions.

KEY TERMS

Intermittent claudication	Pitting edema
Peripheral neuropathy	Varicose veins

Introduction

The peripheral vascular system consists of the portion of the circulatory system that circulates throughout the body, not including the brain or the heart. This system is composed of arteries and veins that transport blood and oxygen throughout the body. This chapter will discuss portions of the peripheral vascular system that are pertinent to the pharmacist.

© antishock/Shutterstock, Inc.

The role of the pharmacist in regard to assessment of the peripheral vascular system can vary greatly depending on the practice setting and the patient's presenting symptoms. Disorders of the peripheral vascular system are referred to as peripheral vascular disease. The key role that a pharmacist can play includes proper triage of patients who may present with new symptoms or worsening symptoms of an established peripheral vascular condition. Because certain diseases can place a patient at higher risk of developing peripheral vascular disease, pharmacists can play a role in screening and educating patients about the peripheral vascular conditions.

Core questions related to symptom onset, location, duration, character, aggravating factors, relieving factors, timing, and severity should be incorporated into the patient interview. Additional questions, which will be discussed further in this chapter, should also be included in the interview depending on the patient's presenting condition.

Components of the Peripheral Vascular Exam

Physical examination for the pharmacist consists primarily of palpation and inspection of parts of the extremities commonly affected by peripheral artery disease or other conditions of the circulatory system. Palpation involves feeling the area to assess changes in skin temperature, quality of the pulse, and presence of edema. Inspection involves viewing the area for changes in skin appearance, presence or absence of body hair, and change of skin color, swelling, or edema.

Clinical Presentation of Symptoms and Disease Processes Related to the Peripheral Vascular System

Peripheral Artery Disease

Peripheral artery disease (PAD) is a type of peripheral vascular disease that typically affects the legs, but can also affect the arms. PAD occurs when atherosclerotic plaques form in the vessels and arteries in the rest of the body, excluding the vasculature of the heart (Hirsch, 2006). These atherosclerotic plaques limit the blood flow to areas of the body. As with patients with coronary artery disease, patients with PAD are also at risk for heart attack and stroke (Hirsch, 2006).

Peripheral artery disease is characterized by cramping and pain in the legs, referred to as **intermittent claudication**. The pain usually affects the thigh, calf, or buttock area. This pain occurs during activity, such as walking or exercise, and resolves with rest; however, in long-standing PAD, the patient may experience pain at rest as well (Hoeben, 2009; Hirsch, 2006; Creager, 2012). Other symptoms of PAD include extremities—usually the legs—that feel cool to the touch and are pale in appearance, and numbness and tingling sensations in the extremity (Creager, 2012). Limb ischemia, in which the blood flow to the extremity is extremely poor, can occur in severe cases of PAD. Patients with limb ischemia may be at risk for gangrene (Hirsch, 2006). Patients presenting with symptoms suggestive of PAD should be referred to their primary care provider.

The Patient Interview

Patients with PAD may initially present complaining of pain in the legs. Because pain can be a symptom of many conditions, the patient interview should include questions that

Intermittent claudication:
A symptom of peripheral artery disease that is characterized by episodes of pain, cramping, and fatigue in one or both legs. It is precipitated by physical exertion and resolves at rest.

can help discern and possibly rule out pain of musculoskeletal origin. In addition, the pharmacist should ask questions that can help determine if the pain is due to a thrombo-embolic process, such as a blood clot, also known as a deep vein thrombosis (DVT; see **Table 10-1**). One of the cardinal symptoms of PAD is intermittent claudication; therefore, the pharmacist should ask the patient if the pain occurs during walking or exercise and resolves with rest. If the pain with activity is recurrent, the pharmacist can also ask how long a patient can perform an activity before the pain occurs. Because coronary artery disease (CAD) is often present in patients with PAD, asking the patient about past medical history of CAD is important. Additionally, asking about the presence of risk factors for PAD is helpful in narrowing down that the pain is possibly the result of PAD (**Table 10-2**).

For those patients with existing PAD that has been diagnosed, the patient interview will vary if the patient is presenting with new symptoms that may be related to PAD. Certainly, the interview should be designed to determine if new pain is due to PAD or another cause. In addition, questions to help best describe the new symptoms should be included. The pharmacist should ask those patients who may be returning to the pharmacy after a drug therapy change for pain associated with PAD, or who are being followed by a pharmacist for medication therapy management, about improvement of symptoms as a result of drug therapy changes.

Table 10-1 Signs and Symptoms of Deep Vein Thrombosis

- Pain or cramping in the affected extremity that lasts for several days with increasing discomfort
- Unilateral swelling and edema surrounding the area of suspected embolus
- Affected area is warm to touch
- Erythema
- Discomfort with palpation of the area

Questions to ask
1. When did the symptoms start?
2. Have the symptoms improved, worsened, or stayed the same since the onset?
3. Have you had any recent travel that required prolonged times of immobility?

Data from Goldhaber SZ. Deep venous thrombosis and pulmonary thromboembolism. In: Longo DL, Fauci AS, Kasper DL, Hauser SL, Jameson J, Loscalzo J, eds. *Harrison's Principles of Internal Medicine*. 18th ed. New York: McGraw-Hill; 2012. Available at: http://accesspharmacy.mhmedical.com/content.aspx?bookid=331&Sectionid=40727045.

Table 10-2 Risk Factors for PAD

African American ethnicity
Age (> 40)
Current cigarette smoking
Diabetes
Hypertension
Hypercholesterolemia
Renal insufficiency

Data from Selvin E, Erlinger T. Prevalence of and risk factors for peripheral arterial disease in the United States: results from the National Health and Nutrition Examination Survey, 1999–2000. *Circulation*. 2004;110:738–743.

Case #1

JB is a 65-year-old man who is managed by the clinical pharmacist at the pharmacotherapy clinic. His past medical history (PMH) is significant for hypertension, diabetes, and hyperlipidemia. He presents today complaining of recurrent pain below the calf area. He states that the pain started about 1 week ago, when he was out walking his dog.

Question

1. What additional questions could you ask JB to help determine if this problem is due to PAD rather than DVT? Why?

The Physical Exam

The pharmacist's physical assessment for PAD is composed of inspection and palpation. It involves comparing the findings of one extremity to the other, and noting differences between the two, as well as differences from what is considered normal. Inspection of the extremity should involve looking for changes in skin color and appearance. In PAD, skin may appear pale and shiny. Inspection should also consist of looking for the presence of wounds or sores that are slow to heal, as well as signs of skin necrosis or gangrene (FIGURE 10-1). In addition, if the patient has hair on the extremity, one should look to determine if there are areas of the extremity where hair appears to be missing (Hirsch, 2006; Bickley, 2009).

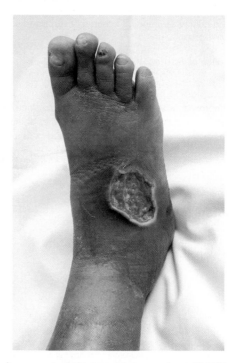

FIGURE 10-1 Slow-healing sores and skin necrosis in a patient with PAD.
© nikolaykaz/iStock/Thinkstock

The next portion of the examination consists of palpation. Palpation should include comparing skin temperature of the extremities (FIGURE 10-2). The extremity affected by PAD may feel cool compared to the other extremity. In addition, one should palpate the dorsalis pedis and tibial pulses. The dosalis pedis pulse is located on the top of the foot (Hirsch, 2006; Bickley, 2009) (FIGURE 10-3), and the tibial pulse is located in the inside

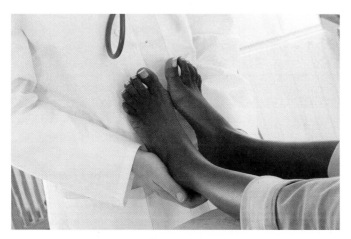

FIGURE 10-2 Comparing skin temperature of the extremities.
© BSIP/Phototake

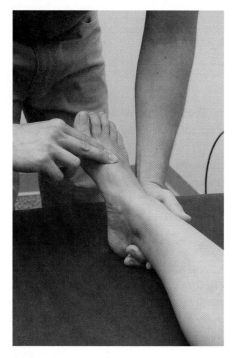

FIGURE 10-3 Palpating the dorsalis pedis pulse.

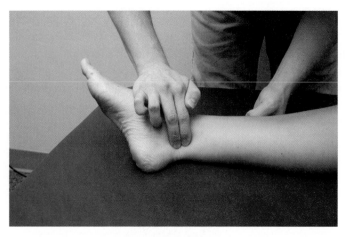

FIGURE 10-4 Palpating the tibial pulse.

of the ankle (**FIGURE 10-4**). The presence of a weak pulse or a pulse that is not palpable can be a sign of PAD (Hirsch, 2006; Bickley, 2009).

Case #1 *(continued)*

Based on JB's responses, you determine that his pain is most likely related to PAD and not DVT.

Question
2. What physical exam findings would be consistent with PAD?

Varicose veins:
Veins that have become twisted and enlarged, and which may be accompanied by pain.

Chronic Venous Insufficiency

Chronic venous insufficiency is a condition of the lower extremities caused by the inability of blood to flow through the veins and back to the heart. This can be due to a blockage in the veins or due to poorly functioning valves in the veins that allow blood to flow backward (Eberhardt, 2005; Weiss, 2012). It is characterized by enlarged veins that appear under the skin on the affected extremity. The veins, also called **varicose veins**, are visible and appear in a twisted formation. Other signs and symptoms include edema, swelling, skin discoloration, and pain. In severe cases, ulcers can form (Eberhardt, 2005; Weiss, 2012). Some risk factors for venous insufficiency are listed in **Table 10-3**. Patients presenting with chronic venous insufficiency should be referred to the primary care provider. However, because one of the treatment options for management of this disorder is the use of compression stockings, some patients may be referred to the pharmacist for compression stocking fittings.

The Patient Interview

A patient with chronic venous insufficiency may present with physical concerns ranging from swelling and pain to cosmetic concerns related to varicose veins. The swelling or pain may cause problems with clothing and shoes not fitting properly. Patients for whom varicose veins is the primary concern may present to the pharmacist asking about methods that can be used to reduce the size or cover up the varicose veins. Regardless of the

Table 10-3 Risk Factors for Venous Insufficiency

Family history
Leg injury
Obesity
Older age
Pregnancy
Prolonged standing
Women

Data from Criqui M, Denenberg J, Bergan J, Langer R, Fronek A. Risk factors for chronic venous disease: the San Diego Population Study. *J Vasc Surg.* 2007;46(2):331–337.

patient's presenting concern, an interview using the core questions should be performed. In addition, inquiry regarding the presence of pain is important.

The Physical Exam

The physical exam for chronic venous insufficiency involves inspecting the lower legs for the presence of varicose veins. The skin should be assessed for hyperpigmentation and the presence of ulcers (**FIGURE 10-5**). The pharmacist should inspect the leg for the presence of edema (Bickley, 2009; Krishnan, 2005). If present, palpation for edema (**FIGURE 10-6**) should be performed to assess the level of edema. Edema can be described as nonpitting edema or **pitting edema**. Edema is characterized as pitting edema if after pressure is applied to the edematous area the skin remains indented, or pitted, where the pressure was applied. In addition, measurement of the circumference of the extremity can be done to determine the amount of edema, because the affected extremity may be larger in circumference compared to the nonaffected extremity (Bickley, 2009).

Pitting edema: Classification for edema in which an impression is left on the affected area when pressed upon.

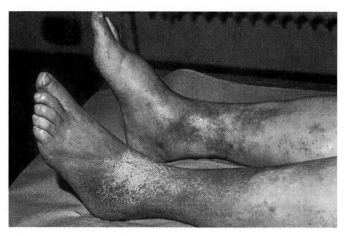

FIGURE 10-5 Hyperpigmentation in a chronic venous insufficiency.
© Watney Collection/Phototake, Inc.

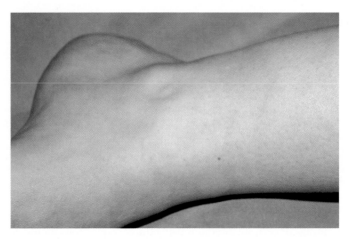

FIGURE 10-6 Pitting edema.
© Jones and Bartlett Publishers. Photographed by Kimberly Potvin.

Vascular Complications of Diabetes:
Peripheral Neuropathy and Diabetic Foot Ulcers

Patients with diabetes, especially those with poorly controlled diabetes, are at risk for developing foot ulcers. According to the American Diabetes Association (ADA) (2014), proper foot care can prevent the development of foot ulcers. Prevention of diabetic foot ulcers is very important in regard to foot care in patients with diabetes. The pharmacist's role in foot care is primarily related to screening and education.

Diabetes can affect both the microvasculature and macrovasculature. Microvascular complications involve the small blood vessels, and can affect the eyes, kidneys, and nerves. **Peripheral neuropathy** is a microvascular condition that affects the nerves in the legs and feet. Macrovascular complications involve the larger blood vessels and can result in peripheral artery disease. Effects of PAD can be manifested in the foot of patients with diabetes.

Peripheral neuropathy that affects the lower extremities can be divided into three categories: motor neuropathy, sensory neuropathy, and Charcot neuropathy (**Table 10-4**).

Because this condition affects the nerves, patients with peripheral neuropathy may experience loss of feeling or sensation in the leg or foot. As a result, the patient may not recognize damage or injury to the extremity.

Peripheral neuropathy:
A condition characterized by nerve damage that presents as sensations of numbness, tingling, and pain in the extremities.

The Patient Interview

Depending on the practice setting, the patient interview for the diabetic foot may have to be initiated by the pharmacist. In some patient care settings, such as clinics or doctors' offices, clinicians require all patients with diabetes to take off shoes and socks at each visit upon entering the exam room. In these settings, the patient will expect that a foot examination will be performed and may wait until the clinician begins the interview. In some cases, the patient may initiate the interview if he or she has noticed sores or other problems with the foot. In a community pharmacy setting, on the other hand, patients may not expect the pharmacist to inquire about foot care; therefore, performing a patient interview in regard to foot care may be awkward. Because the ADA (2014) recommends that persons with diabetes check their

Table 10-4 Comparison of Peripheral Neuropathies

	Motor Neuropathy	Sensory Neuropathy	Charcot Neuropathy
Which nerves are affected?	Nerves that innervate the muscles	Nerves that innervate the toes, legs, and hands	Nerves that innervate the bones and joints of the foot
Clinical presentation	Muscle atrophy and muscle weakness	Pain and burning sensations in the extremities; tingling and aching at night	Stress fractures
Result	Alterations in walking patterns due to foot deformities, which leads to the development of calluses and foot ulcers	Alterations in sensation related to pain, pressure, and temperature, which can lead to injury and ultimately development of foot ulcers	Severe foot deformity due to inability to sense pain from fractures; bone regrowth leads to deformities, which leads to the development of ulcers

Data from Holt P. Assessment and management of patients with diabetic foot ulcers. *Nurs Stand*. 2013;27:49–55.

feet daily as a part of their normal hygiene routine, a good way to start an interview in this setting could be by saying, "I notice that you have diabetes. Can you tell me how often you check your feet for sores, cuts, or injuries?" In other instances, the interview may be initiated as a result of a patient presenting with a complaint. Regardless of how the interview is started, key information that should be ascertained includes how often the patient performs foot inspections, if the patient has noticed new or worsening pain or loss of sensation, if the patient has noticed any sores that are slow to heal, and if the patient has noticed any new signs of infection (ADA, 2014; Boulton, 2008). The presence of any of these factors should warrant a recommendation to the patient's primary care provider. In addition, the pharmacist should ask whether the patient has a history of ulcers or amputations (ADA, 2014; Boulton, 2008).

The Physical Exam

The physical examination of the foot involves inspecting the foot for the presence of deformity, calluses, ulcers, and infection. In addition, the foot should be inspected for areas of redness and swelling, which may suggest an area of recent injury or an area where a callus may form. The inspection should not be limited to the surface areas of the feet. The inspection should also involve looking in between the toes and under the toes if the patient's toes tend to curl under. The toenails should also be inspected for signs of damage, change in color, and change in toenail thickness (Boulton, 2008).

Shoes should be inspected as well for signs of uneven wear, which can be a sign of altered walking patterns. Additionally shoes should be assessed to determine if they may be too small or too narrow for the patient's foot, which can contribute to the development of calluses. Finally, socks should be inspected for the presence of blood or fluid that may suggest injury or infection (Boulton, 2008).

The foot should also be assessed for the presence or absence of sensations (ADA, 2014; Boulton, 2008). This can be done using the monofilament test (**FIGURE 10-7**). This test involves touching various areas of the foot to see if the patient feels the sensation. The patient then reports if he or she felt the sensation. Examination of the foot should

Self Testing Instructions

(You may screen your own feet or ask a relative, friend, or neighbor to do it for you)

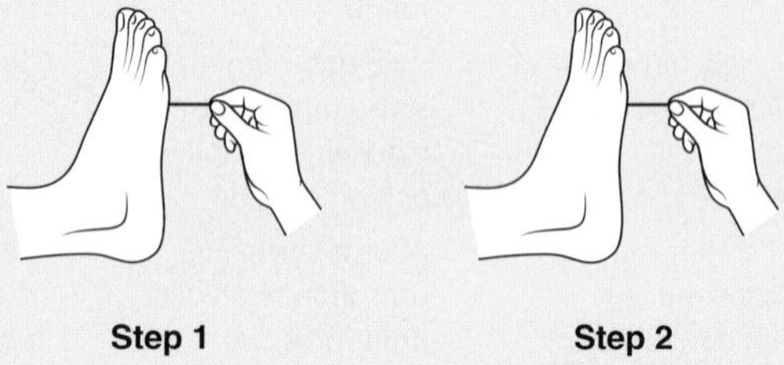

Step 1   Step 2

1. Hold the red filament by the paper handle, as shown in Step 1.
2. Use a smooth motion to touch the filament to the skin on your foot. Touch the filament along the side of and NOT directly on an ulcer, callous, or scar. Touch the filament to your skin for 1-2 seconds. Push hard enough to make the filament bend as shown in Step 2.
3. Touch the filament to both of your feet in the sites circled on the drawing below.
4. Place a (+) in the circle if you can feel the filament at that site and a (−) if you cannot feel the filament at that site.
5. The filament is reusable. After use, wipe with an alcohol swab.

Foot Screen Test Sites

If you have a (−) in any circle, take this form to your healthcare provider as soon as possible.

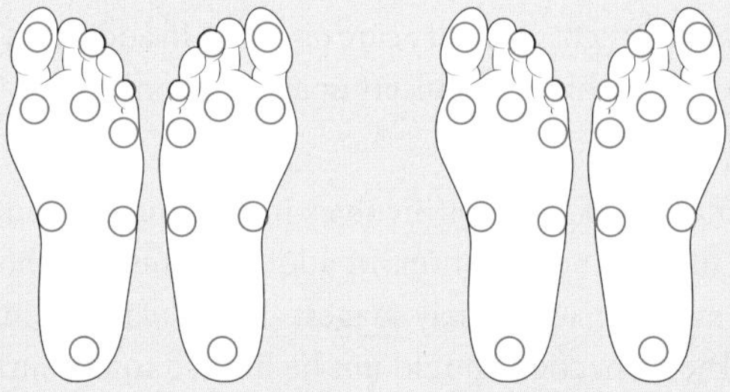

Date _____   Date _____

Place Filament Here

FIGURE 10-7 Diabetic foot screen for sensation.

Reproduced from National Hansen's Disease Programs, LEAP Program, 1770 Physicians Park Dr., Baton Rouge, LA 70816.

also include palpation of the dorsalis pedis and tibial pulses to determine the presence or absence of a pulse. Finally, the temperature of the foot should be assessed in comparison to the other foot and other areas of the leg (Boulton, 2008).

Findings from the foot examination can help determine the patient's foot risk category. **Table 10-5** defines the risk categories, treatment options, and the pharmacist's role in triage.

Table 10-5 Foot Risk Categories

Risk Category	Definition	Pharmacist's Triage Recommendations
Low Risk Category 0	Patient has no deformities, has all sensations in foot, no amputations or foot ulcers, no peripheral artery disease	Notify primary care provider Suggest annual foot examination Provide patient education on proper foot care
High Risk		
High Risk Category 1	Lost sensations in foot *and/or* presence of deformity	Refer patient to Primary Care provider for further examination
High Risk Category 2	Lost sensations in foot *and/or* peripheral artery disease	Suggest annual foot examination
High Risk Category 3	History of amputation or foot ulcers	Provide patient education on proper foot care

Modified from Boulton A, Armstrong D, Albert S. Frykberg R, Hellman R, Kirkman M. Comprehensive foot examination and risk assessment. A report of the task force of the foot care interest group of the American Diabetes Association, with endorsement by the American Association of Clinical Endocrinologists. *Diabetes Care*. 2008;31:1679–1685.

Clinical Presentation of Drug-Induced Processes

Drug-Induced Peripheral Edema

When evaluating a patient with edema, it is important to include a review of the patient's medication list in the evaluation process. A number of medications have been implicated in causing peripheral edema (**Table 10-6**).

The patient interview should include questions designed to help determine a temporal relationship between when the drug was started and when the edema appeared.

Table 10-6 Medications That Can Cause Peripheral Edema

Amlodipine
Felodipine
Gabapentin
Nifedipine
Pioglitazone
Pregabalin

Data from Drugs that commonly cause peripheral edema. *Pharmacist's Letter/Prescriber's Letter*. 2011;27(9):270918.

Case #2

You are participating in a diabetes foot screening awareness day at a local community center. You are preparing to perform a monofilament test on LH, a 68-year-old man with type 2 diabetes, PAD, hypertension, and hyperlipidemia.

Question

1. What questions would you like to ask LH to assess for the presence of peripheral neuropathy prior to examining his feet?

Case #2 *(continued)*

LH tells you that he has not noticed any sores on his feet that have been slow to heal and has not noticed any pain. While performing the test, you determine that LH has lost sensation in his left big toe, as well as in his left and right heels. You also notice that his tibial and dorsalis pedis pulses are weak, and the skin temperature of his left foot and leg feels slightly cooler than that of the right leg.

Question

2. Based on your findings, what is LH's foot risk? What would be your recommendation to LH?

Cultural Considerations with the Peripheral Vascular System

Although literature discussing the use of explanatory models with patients with peripheral vascular conditions is lacking, the use of these models may be helpful for the pharmacist when providing patient care. As done with other medication conditions, allowing the patient to explain his or her beliefs about the condition and how to treat it can provide useful information. In addition, use of explanatory models may help the pharmacist learn more about the patient's risk factors for disease of the peripheral vascular system, the patient's knowledge level about the condition, and healthcare practices.

Pharmacists should also be aware of the presence of a disparity in the rate of lower extremity amputations in patients with diabetes. Diabetes has been noted by the Centers for Disease Control and Prevention to be the leading cause of nontraumatic amputations (CDC, 2011). Reducing the rate of lower extremity amputations in patients diagnosed with diabetes has been identified as an objective by Healthy People 2020. Pharmacists can play a role in addressing this disparity by implementing proactive screening and educational initiatives that will help address the goals of Healthy People 2020.

One major preventative factor that can potentially contribute to the reduction of amputations and health disparities is performing self-care behaviors related to foot care. Educating the patient on self-care is an important role that the pharmacist can play. However, as was discovered in studies by Nwasuruba et al. (2007) and Olson et al. (2009), ethnic differences in foot care behaviors and basic knowledge regarding foot care can be present within the patient population. The use of an explanatory model during the information-gathering portion of the patient interview can help the pharmacist learn about those behaviors that are specific to the individual patient, and therefore allow him or her to provide customized education.

Summary

There are many opportunities for a pharmacist to play an integral role in the screening and management of peripheral vascular conditions. Through patient interview and physical examination the pharmacist can help to identify patients at risk for peripheral artery disease and refer patients for proper treatment upon discovery of PAD complications. Certain patient populations experience a disproportionate rate of lower extremity amputations. Pharmacists, who are highly accessible to the community, can help to identify and refer patients at risk for amputation to other healthcare providers and provide education to the patient as a means to prevent further complications.

Review Questions

1. Compare and contrast the difference in clinical presentation between venous insufficiency and PAD.
2. While you are working at the community pharmacy, a 50-year-old woman approaches the counter to ask for advice regarding her swollen ankles. The patient states that she noticed the swelling for the past month, but it seems to have worsened over the past 2 weeks. The patient's medical history is significant for hypertension, hyperlipidemia, and arthritis. Her medication history is as follows:

Rx Number	Medication	Last Date Filled
106282	Ibuprofen 800 mg po TID	1 month ago
106257	Amlodipine 10 mg po QD	2 weeks ago
105258	HCTZ 25 mg po QD	1 month ago
105257	Amlodipine 5 mg po QD	1 month ago

Based on her medication profile, which medication(s) are most likely contributing to her edema?

References

American Diabetes Association. Foot Care. Available at: http://www.diabetes.org/living-with-diabetes/complications/foot-complications/foot-care.html. Updated March 11, 2014. Accessed August 23, 2014.

American Diabetes Association. Standards of medical care in diabetes—2014. *Diabetes Care.* 2014;37(suppl1):S14–S80.

Bickley L, Szilagyi P. The peripheral vascular system. In: Bickley L, Szilagyi P, eds. *Bates' Guide to Physical Examination and History Taking.* 10th ed. Philadelphia, PA: Lippincott Williams & Wilkins; 2009;471–499.

Boulton A, Armstrong D, Albert S, Frykberg R, Hellman R, Kirkman M. Comprehensive foot examination and risk assessment. A report of the Task Force of the Foot Care Interest Group of the American Diabetes Association, with endorsement by the American Association of Clinical Endocrinologists. *Diabetes Care.* 2008;31:1679–1685.

Centers for Disease Control and Prevention. *National Diabetes Fact Sheet: National Estimates and General Information on Diabetes and Prediabetes in the United States, 2011.* Atlanta, GA: U.S. Department of Health and Human Services, Centers for Disease Control and Prevention; 2011. Available at: http://www.cdc.gov/diabetes/pubs/pdf/ndfs_2011.pdf. Accessed August 21, 2013.

Creager M, Loscalzo J. Vascular diseases of the extremities. In: Fauci AS, Kasper DL, Jameson JL, Longo DL, Hauser SL, eds. *Harrison's Principles of Internal Medicine.* 18th ed. New York: McGraw-Hill; 2012. Available at: http://accesspharmacy.mhmedical.com.bluestem.csu.edu:2048/content.aspx?bookid=331&sectionid=40727028. Accessed August 23, 2014.

Criqui M, Denenberg J, Bergan J, Langer R, Fronek A. Risk factors for chronic venous disease: the San Diego Population Study. *J Vasc Surg.* 2007;46(2):331–337.

Drugs that commonly cause peripheral edema. *Pharmacist's Letter/Prescriber's Letter* 2011;27(9):270918.

Eberhardt R, Raffetto J. Chronic venous insufficiency. *Circulation*. 2005;111:2398–2409.

Goldhaber SZ. Deep venous thrombosis and pulmonary thromboembolism. In: Fauci AS, Kasper DL, Jameson JL, Longo DL, Hauser SL, eds. *Harrison's Principles of Internal Medicine*. 18th ed. New York: McGraw-Hill; 2012. Available at: http://www.accesspharmacy.com/content.aspx?aID=9128812. Accessed April 30, 2013.

Healthy People.gov. 2020 topics and objectives. Diabetes. Available at: http://www.healthypeople.gov/2020/topicsobjectives2020/overview.aspx?topicId=8. Accessed April 29, 2013.

Hirsch A, Haskal Z, Hertzer N, Bakal C, Creager M, Halpern J, et al. ACC/AHA 2005 guidelines for the management of patients with peripheral arterial disease (lower extremity, renal, mesenteric, and abdominal aortic): Executive summary a collaborative report from the American Association for Vascular Surgery/Society for Vascular Surgery, Society for Cardiovascular Angiography and Interventions, Society for Vascular Medicine and Biology, Society of Interventional Radiology, and the ACC/AHA Task Force on Practice Guidelines (Writing Committee to Develop Guidelines for the Management of Patients With Peripheral Arterial Disease). *J Am Coll Cardiol*. 2006;47(6):1239–1312.

Hoeben BJ. Peripheral arterial disease. In: Wofford MR, Posey LM, Linn WD, O'Keefe ME, eds. *Pharmacotherapy in Primary Care*. New York: McGraw-Hill; 2009. Available at: http://www.accesspharmacy.com/content.aspx?aID=3601480. Accessed April 30, 2013.

Holt P. Assessment and management of patients with diabetic foot ulcers. *Nurs Stand*. 2013;27:49–55.

Krishnan S, Nicholls S. Chronic venous insufficiency: clinical assessment and patient selection. *Semin Intervent Radiol*. 2005;22(3):169–177.

Nwasuruba C, Khan M, Egede L. Racial/ethnic differences in multiple self-care behaviors in adults with diabetes. *J Gen Intern Med*. 2007;22:115–120.

Olson J, Hogan M, Pogach L, Rajan M, Raugi G, Reiber G. Foot care education and self management behaviors in diverse veterans with diabetes. *Patient Prefer Adherence*. 2009;3:45–50.

Selvin E, Erlinger T. Prevalence of and risk factors for peripheral arterial disease in the United States: results from the National Health and Nutrition Examination Survey, 1999–2000. *Circulation*. 2004;110:738–743.

Weiss R, Izaguirre D, Lanza J, Klaus-Dieter L. Venous insufficiency. Medscape. Available at: http://emedicine.medscape.com/article/1085412-overview. Updated November 21, 2012. Accessed August 23, 2014.

Chapter 11

Musculoskeletal Assessment
Yolanda M. Hardy, PharmD

LEARNING OBJECTIVES

At the completion of this chapter, the reader should be able to:

1. Determine appropriate questions to ask patients when performing a focused musculoskeletal system interview.

2. Explain the clinical presentation of common symptoms and diseases related to the musculoskeletal system.

3. Explain how to correctly perform the physical assessment techniques related to the musculoskeletal system.

4. List medications that can cause adverse effects or medical conditions affecting the musculoskeletal system.

5. Explain the clinical presentation of drug-induced disease processes.

6. Triage patients based on clinical presentation of problems related to the musculoskeletal system.

7. Explain cultural concepts regarding pain and pain management.

KEY TERMS

Acute	Localized	Rhabdomyolysis
Chronic	Myalgia	Sprain
Generalized	Myositis	Strain

Introduction

Conditions related to the musculoskeletal system can involve bones, joints, tendons, or muscles. These conditions can be **acute**, in which the onset is short and the condition is relatively temporary, or **chronic**, in which the condition is present over a long period of time. In addition, musculoskeletal conditions can be **localized**, affecting only a small, specific area of the body, or **generalized**, affecting a larger area of the body or potentially the entire body. These conditions can be precipitated by injury, overuse of a muscle, or

© antishock/Shutterstock, Inc.

Acute:
A condition with sudden onset that may resolve with or without treatment.

Chronic:
A condition that presents and lasts for a long period of time. The condition may involve continuous symptoms or may present with intermittent symptoms.

Localized:
Describes symptoms that are limited to one particular area of the body or organ system.

Generalized:
Describes symptoms that are not limited to one particular area of the body or organ system. Symptoms may affect the entire body.

a medical condition. The symptoms of musculoskeletal conditions, regardless of their origin, are similar. Pain, swelling, muscle weakness, and fatigue are common symptoms; however, these symptoms are also present in conditions that are nonmusculoskeletal in origin. Although the pharmacist is not in the role of making diagnoses, the assessment performed should involve determining if the symptoms the patient is experiencing are due to musculoskeletal problems, if the problem is acute or chronic, and whether the patient's condition is able to be treated with or without referral to a primary care provider or an emergency care provider.

Pain is one of the common presenting symptoms of musculoskeletal problems. In addition, musculoskeletal problems can occur in any area of the body. Taking this into consideration, the pharmacist should be aware of and highly sensitive to complaints of pain located in the chest. Chest pain can be the result of multiple conditions, ranging from a minor muscle strain to a more serious condition such as a myocardial infarction or pulmonary embolism (Karnath, 2004). As a result, complaints of chest pain should be assessed quickly (**Table 11-1**) so that proper care can be provided in an efficient manner.

The pharmacist's assessment of the musculoskeletal system is performed primarily through patient interview; however, in some instances performing a physical exam that involves inspection and palpation of the affected area can provide more information needed to make a decision. Assessment of musculoskeletal conditions via interview and physical exam can help the pharmacist determine if the patient can treat the condition with or without referral to the primary care provider, or whether he or she should seek emergent help.

For an acute condition, the patient interview should incorporate the core questions related to symptom onset, location, duration, character, aggravating factors, relieving factors, timing, and severity for acute conditions, such as injury. For chronic diseases, questions that will help determine worsening of symptoms compared to baseline are important. Musculoskeletal conditions can result in limited range of motion of the affected body part and can prevent the patient from performing daily activities.

Case #1

PA is a 36-year-old man who presents to the pharmacy seeking a recommendation for pain. He states that 2 weeks ago he was diagnosed with high cholesterol, and in order to make lifestyle changes he joined a weekend softball team for exercise. Yesterday was PA's first practice with the team. He states that during practice he did pushups with the team and also practiced throwing and catching the softball. PA tells you that this morning he woke up with pain in his chest, left shoulder, and left arm. He also states that he thinks his left arm feels weak. He states that although it has been over a year since he has exercised, he has never experienced this feeling before.

Questions
1. What additional questions would you ask PA to determine if his chest pain is musculoskeletal in origin?
2. Is PA's complaint consistent with a musculoskeletal injury? Why?
3. Would you consider PA's condition acute or chronic? Why?

Table 11-1 Differentiating Types of Chest Pain

Source of Pain	Causes	Pain Assessment	Treatment
Chest pain of musculo-skeletal origin	Inflammation of costochondroids Injury	Localized to the chest wall area. Palpation of affected area may reproduce the pain; pain may be present upon movement. Patient will usually point to the area with index finger.	May be treated with self-care measures; severe pain or pain that limits performance of daily activities should be further assessed by a primary care provider.
Chest pain due to herpes zoster (shingles)	Activation of herpes zoster	Described as burning pain over dermatomes. Vesicular lesions may or may not be present.	Requires referral to primary care provider for initial assessment and treatment. May be managed with self-care measures under the advice of the primary care provider.
Chest pain of cardiac origin	Angina	Described as heavy pressure or squeezing.	Requires prompt referral to primary care provider. Severe symptoms may require immediate care in an acute care setting.
	Myocardial infarction	Accompanied by sweating, nausea, vomiting, and weakness. Patient may physically clench fist over sternum when describing pain.	Requires immediate care in an acute care setting.
	Aortic stenosis	Described as occurring with activity.	Requires prompt referral to primary care provider. Severe symptoms may require immediate care in an acute care setting.
	Coronary vasospasm	Similar pain as angina; however, pain occurs mostly at rest instead of during activity.	Requires prompt referral to primary care provider. Severe symptoms may require immediate care in an acute care setting.
	Cardiomyopathy	Similar pain as angina; however, patient may also present with dyspnea and/or syncope.	Requires prompt referral to primary care provider. Severe symptoms may require immediate care in an acute care setting.
	Pericarditis	Describes pleuritic pain that is relieved by sitting forward and worsened by lying down.	Requires prompt referral to primary care provider. Severe symptoms may require immediate care in an acute care setting.

(continues)

Table 11-1 Differentiating Types of Chest Pain (*continued*)

Source of Pain	Causes	Pain Assessment	Treatment
	Aortic aneurism	Describes pain as originating in the front of the chest and radiating to the upper back.	Requires prompt referral to primary care provider. Severe symptoms may require immediate care in an acute care setting.
	Mitral valve prolapse	Described as sharp pain over the bottom-most part of the heart (apex). Pain is relieved or minimized by lying down.	Requires prompt referral to primary care provider. Severe symptoms may require immediate care in an acute care setting.
Chest pain of gastro-intestinal origin	Esophageal spasm	Described as pain that occurs with swallowing hot or cold substances.	Requires prompt referral to primary care provider. Severe symptoms may require immediate care in an acute care setting.
	Esophageal perforation	Described as constant pain in the neck to the epigastrium. Worsens with swallowing.	Requires prompt referral to primary care provider. Severe symptoms may require immediate care in an acute care setting.
	Esophageal reflux	Described as a burning sensation. May worsen after meals or when lying down.	Mild cases may be treated with self-care methods.
	Esophagitis	Described as chest pain and pain with swallowing.	Mild cases may be treated with self-care methods.
Chest pain of pulmonary origin	Pluritic conditions	Described as sharp. Worsens with coughing, deep breathing, or movement.	Requires prompt referral to primary care provider.
	Pneumothorax	Described as sharp pain that radiates to the shoulder on the same side of the body.	Requires immediate care in an acute care setting.
	Pulmonary embolism	Described as pleuritic chest pain, accompanied by dyspnea and hypoxia.	Requires immediate care in an acute care setting.

Data from Karnath B, Holden M, Hussain N. Chest pain: differentiating cardiac from noncardiac causes. *Hosp Physician.* 2004;38:24–27.

Clinical Presentation of Symptoms and Disease Processes Related to the Musculoskeletal System

Acute Musculoskeletal Conditions

Acute muscle injury can be the result of muscle **sprain**, when the ligament tears or stretches, or **strain**, when the muscle or tendon stretches or tears due to performing physical activity or lifting objects. A sprain or strain can also occur as the result of loss of balance or performing repetitive motions. These acute muscle injuries can affect any muscle in the body, but most commonly affect the elbows, ankles, or hamstrings. Symptoms of muscle strain include pain at rest or during use of the muscle, bruising, and muscle weakness. In some instances the patient may not be able to move the affected muscle. Muscle sprains can cause pain, inflammation and warmth near the joint, and bruising. Sprains and strains can be treated using self-care measures; however, note that many of the symptoms of sprains and strains are similar to those for fractures, which require medical treatment (**FIGURE 11-1**).

> **Sprain:**
> An injury resulting from stretching or tearing of ligaments.

> **Strain:**
> An injury resulting from stretching or tearing of muscle or tendons.

Muscle overuse injuries can result from performing repetitive movements of a limb (Chumbley, 2000). This type of injury can occur in people who participate in sports such as tennis, swimming, golf, or weight lifting. The injury occurs as a result of irritation to the tendons or muscle affected by the repetitive activity. Continuation of the activity without treating the injury can lead to damage, including tendon rupture (Chumbley, 2000). Most overuse injuries can be treated using self-care measures; however, serious cases warrant referral to a primary care provider.

The Patient Interview

The patient interview should include questioning about what activities the patient was doing prior to experiencing the pain. In addition, the patient should be asked if the symptoms occur only when active or performing a particular activity, or whether they also occur at rest.

The Physical Exam

A pharmacist can perform a limited physical assessment that includes inspection of the affected area to complement findings from the patient interview. The physical exam can

---

"Is It Broken?"

Suspect a bone fracture if:
1) Affected area shows deformity.
2) Pain worsens upon movement or when pressure is applied.
3) There is a loss of function.
4) A portion of the bone has come through the skin.

FIGURE 11-1 Is it broken?

Data from American Academy of Orthopedic Surgeons. Fractures. Available at http://orthoinfo.aaos.org/topic. cfm?topic=A00139. Accessed August 11, 2013 and American Academy of Orthopedic Surgeons. Fractures. Available at www.orthoinfo.aaos.org/topic.cfm?topic=A002524. Accessed May 16, 2014.

also include a visual assessment of range of motion, which can be done by asking the patient if he or she can move the affected area, and then assessing any limitations (Bickley, 2009) (**FIGURE 11-2A** and **11-2B**). If the patient is in too much pain, or if there is concern that further movement could cause further injury, this assessment can be omitted. In this case, simply asking the patient if he or she can move the area would be sufficient.

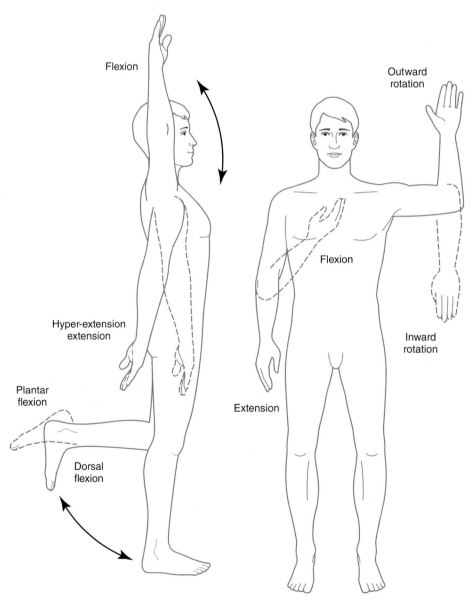

FIGURE 11-2A Range of motion.

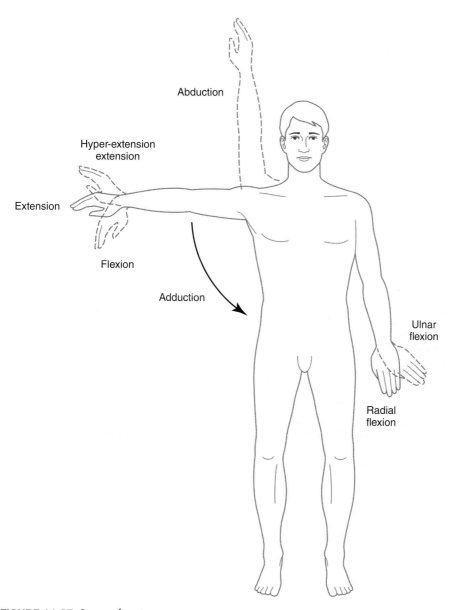

Abduction

Hyper-extension
extension

Extension

Flexion

Adduction

Ulnar
flexion

Radial
flexion

FIGURE 11-2B Range of motion.

Chronic Musculoskeletal Conditions

Arthritis

Arthritis describes disease states that affect the joints. Common conditions that fall under this category include osteoarthritis, rheumatoid arthritis, gout, and septic arthritis (**Table 11-2**). Although patients typically say "arthritis," when they are referring to osteoarthritis, it is important to clarify with the patient the condition they are referring to, rather than assume that the patient means osteoarthritis.

Table 11-2 Comparison Among Types of Arthritis

	Osteoarthritis	Rheumatoid Arthritis	Gouty Arthritis
Presenting Symptoms	Joint stiffness Morning joint stiffness that resolves within 30 minutes Joint pain that worsens with activity Swelling or warmth of the joint Loss of range of motion of the joint	Joint stiffness Morning stiffness that lasts > 60 minutes Joint pain Joint swelling Joint warmth	Joint pain Joint swelling that increases and peaks within 24–48 hours
Risk Factors	Female Past trauma Age Obesity	Older age Family history Smoker	Elderly men and postmenopausal women High purine diet Alcohol use Diuretics Reduced renal clearance Obesity
Affected Areas	Hands Knees Hips Spine Asymmetric joint presentation	Wrists Phalanges Symmetric joint presentation	First metatarsophalangeal joint (big toe) Ankle Knee Asymmetric joint presentation
Treatment	Nonpharmacological Pharmacological Complementary Surgical	Prescription medications	Pharmacotherapy aimed at immediate treatment of current episodes and prevention of future episodes

Data from Davis J, Matteson E. My treatment approach to rheumatoid arthritis. *Mayo Clin Proc.* 2012;87:659–673; Eggebeen A. Gout: an update. *Am Fam Physician.* 2007;76:801–808, 811–812; Sinusas K. Osteoarthritis: diagnosis and treatment. *Am Fam Physician.* 2012;85:49–56; Wasserman A. Diagnosis and management of rheumatoid arthritis. *Am Fam Physician.* 2011;84:1245–1252.

Osteoarthritis (OA) is the most common arthritic condition. It is a disease caused by degeneration of the cartilage in the joints. This condition can occur as a result of overuse of the particular joint, thus causing the cartilage to wear down, or it can be caused by joint injury. Osteoarthritis commonly affects the hand, knee, hip, foot, shoulder, or spine, and may affect one or multiple joints in the body (Sinusas, 2012).

Rheumatoid arthritis (RA) is an autoimmune disorder that affects the joints. The inflammatory response triggered in RA ultimately leads to damage of the cartilage. RA is a chronic condition that affects the hands and wrists most often, and typically affects multiple joints. Patients with RA may also present with systemic symptoms of fatigue, weight loss, and low grade fevers (Wasserman, 2011).

Gouty arthritis is a metabolic disease caused by accumulation and deposition of urate crystals in the joints. Gouty arthritis can be either acute or chronic in nature. Acute gout can be triggered by a diet high in purines, trauma, alcohol use, or medications that increase uric acid levels (Eggebeen, 2007).

The Patient Interview

The patient interview for assessment of arthritis varies slightly depending on the type of arthritis and if the problem is of new onset or a chronic condition. Once it is determined that the patient is experiencing arthritic-type pain, the pharmacist should begin to ask questions that would help determine if the arthritic pain is due to osteoarthritis, rheumatoid arthritis, gout, or another condition. This information is helpful not for diagnostic purposes, because the pharmacist does not diagnose conditions, but so that the pharmacist can determine the best method for patient triage. For a patient who is presenting with symptoms suggestive of arthritis for the first time, use of the core questions will be helpful in determining the problem and proper follow-up. Questions should include a determination of the location of the pain and swelling, as well as the presence of additional symptoms such as fever and malaise. For a patient who has been diagnosed

---

Case #1 *(continued)*

You determine that you should gather more information about PA's pain using the core questions.

4. What additional questions would you ask PA to further assess his concern?

Core Questions	
Onset	
Location	
Duration	
Character	
Aggravating Factors	
Relieving Factors	
Timing	
Severity	

You assess PA's range of motion in his shoulder and arm. Although he experiences some pain and weakness, he is able to move both the arm and shoulder through their full range of motion.

Questions

5. What physical exam observations could you make to determine if PA's chest pain is musculoskeletal?
6. You were able to determine that PA's chest pain is musculoskeletal in origin. Based on your interview and physical exam, could PA treat his condition using self-care measures?

Case #2

IC is a 60-year-old woman whom you regularly see for diabetes education. Today, prior to ending her visit with you, she tells you that for the past 5 months she has been experiencing pain and joint stiffness in her index and ring fingers on her right hand. IC is currently a data entry specialist, and has worked in this position for 40 years. Her job requires her to consistently use her right hand to enter numbers into a calculator. She also mentions to you that when she was a young girl she broke her right index finger

when she accidentally slammed the car door shut on it. IC is worried about these symptoms, because both of her sisters and her mother have rheumatoid arthritis.

Questions

1. Is IC's complaint consistent with a musculoskeletal condition? Why?
2. Would you consider IC's condition acute or chronic? Why?

already, it is important to determine if the problem has worsened. For both instances, one should ask how or if the symptoms are affecting their ability to perform activities of daily living. Assessment of pain using a pain scale is also important (**FIGURE 11-3A** and **11-3B**).

Pain Scales

Pain scales can assist in quantifying the intensity level of a patient's pain.

Numeric Rating Scale
- This is an 11-item scale in which the patient can rank their pain from a score of 0, which is no pain at all, to 10, which is the worst pain imaginable.
- This scale can be administered visually or verbally.

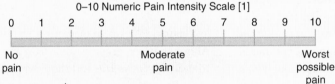

FIGURE 11-3A Numeric rating scale.

Reproduced from Adult Pain Management: Operative Procedures. Quick Reference Guide for Clinicians 1a. Agency for Health Care Policy and Research [now: Agency for Healthcare Research and Quality] Publication No. 92-0019. Rockville, MD; February 1992. (Accessible at http://www.ncbi.nlm.nih.gov/books/NBK52130/).

Wong-Baker FACES Pain Rating Scale
- This is a six-item scale in which the patient can rank pain by selecting from facial expressions that closely resemble how he or she feels regarding the pain.
- Good tool to use when assessing pain in children.

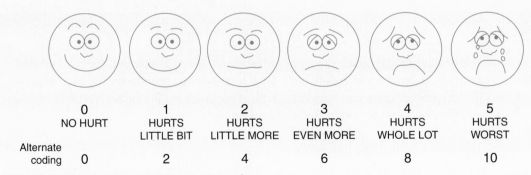

FIGURE 11-3B Wong-Baker FACES pain rating scale.

Reproduced from Hockenberry MJ, Wilson D. *Wong's Essentials of Pediatric Nursing*, 8th ed. St. Louis: Mosby; 2009. Used with permission. Copyright Mosby.

The Physical Exam

In most cases, a pharmacist can perform a limited physical assessment that includes inspection of the affected area to complement findings from the patient interview. The pharmacist can inspect the area of concern for the presence of *nodules or deformities* on or near the affected joints as a result of the disease process. Patients with severe osteoarthritis affecting the hand may present with abnormalities in the hand structure. Heberden nodes are growths that can be seen on the distal interphalangeal (DIP) joint of the osteoarthritic hand. These joints are located at the end of the fingers (Sinusas, 2012). Another structural change that can be seen in the osteoarthritic hand is Bouchard nodes, which are growths seen on the proximal interphalangeal (PIP) joints. These joints are located in the middle of the fingers (Sinusas, 2012). Patients with osteoarthritis of the knee may present with a popliteal cyst, also referred to as a Baker cyst, located in the back of the knee.

Patients with RA may have symmetric deformity in the PIP, metacarpophalangeal (MCP), and wrist joints (Davis, 2012; Wasserman, 2011). These deformities can progress to severe forms that can limit the functionality of the extremity. Chronic RA patients may experience ulnar deviation, in which the fingers of the affected hand shift toward the side or fifth digit of hand. The presence of swan neck deformity or Boutonnière deformity (**FIGURES 11-4A** and **11-4B**) may also be seen in RA. Both the swan neck

---

Case #2 *(continued)*

You determine that you should gather more information about IC's pain using the core questions.

Questions

3. What questions could you ask IC to further determine if her symptoms are due to rheumatoid arthritis?

Core Questions	
Onset	
Location	
Duration	
Character	
Aggravating Factors	
Relieving Factors	
Timing	
Severity	

4. What additional questions would you ask IC to further assess her concern?

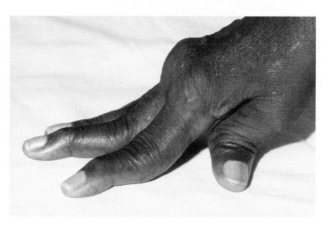

FIGURE 11-4A Swan neck deformity.

© Sue Ford/Science Source

deformity and Boutonnière deformity prevent the finger from being in a straightened position (Bickley, 2009).

The pharmacist can also inspect the area for *swelling and redness*. Redness over the joint could suggest RA or gouty arthritis (Wasserman, 2011; Eggebeen, 2007). Patients experiencing gout attacks will present with swelling and redness over the affected joint (**FIGURE 11-5**).

Patients with new onset of arthritic symptoms or worsening symptoms should be referred for further help from their primary care provider.

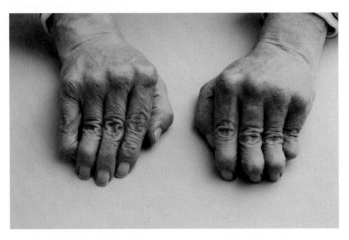

FIGURE 11-4B Boutonnière deformity.
© SPL/Science Source

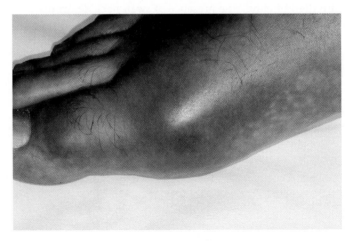

FIGURE 11-5 Foot of patient experiencing a gout attack.
© Dr. P. Marazzi/Science Source

Clinical Presentation of Drug-Induced Processes

Drug-Related Arthritic Conditions

When a patient presents with symptoms suggestive of gout, it is important to review the patient's medication list. A number of medications have been identified as causing arthritis conditions such as gout and pseudogout (**Table 11-3**). Pseudogout is a condition that has a clinical presentation similar to gout; however, it is caused by an accumulation of calcium pyrophosphate salts in the joint rather than an accumulation of urate crystals (Bannwarth, 2007).

> **Case #2** *(continued)*
>
> *Questions*
> 5. What physical exam observations could you make to determine if IC could possibly have signs of arthritis?
> 6. You were able to determine that IC's presentation is more suggestive of osteoarthritis and not rheumatoid arthritis. Based on your interview and physical exam, could IC treat her condition using self-care measures?

Table 11-3 Medications That Can Cause Gout and Pseudogout

Cyanocobalamin	Cyclosporine	Gemfibrozil	H2 blockers
Loop diuretics	Nicotinic acid	Proton pump inhibitors	Tacrolimus
Thiamine	Thiazide diuretics	Bisphosphonates	

Data from Bannwarth B. Drug-induced musculoskeletal disorders. *Drug Safety*. 2007;30:27–46; Bannwarth B. Drug-induced rheumatic disorders. *Rev Rhum Engl Ed*. 1996;63:639–647; Drugs that should be considered potential culprits in patients who present with musculoskeletal disorders. *Drugs Ther Perspect*. 2007;23:21–25; Vergne P, Bertin P, Bonnet C, Scotto C, Treves R. Drug-induced rheumatic disorders: incidence, prevention and management. *Drug Saf*. 2000;23:279–293.

Drug-Related Myopathies

Myopathies, or diseases of the muscles, related to medication use should be considered when assessing a patient with musculoskeletal pain. Drug-induced myopathy can include muscle pain (**myalgia**), muscle inflammation (**myositis**), or **rhabdomyolysis**, which is the breakdown of muscle. If suspected, rhabdomyolysis should be treated immediately. Its clinical presentation includes muscle pain and weakness along with dark-colored urine, described as tea-colored or darker (Huerta-Alardin, 2005; Sathasivam, 2008; Warren, 2002).

Drug-induced rhabdomyolysis should be a part of the workup for a patient presenting with symptoms of muscle pain and weakness due to a cause that cannot be determined or if the patient is currently on a medication that has been associated with rhabdomyolysis (**Table 11-4**). Pharmacists should inquire about the presence or absence of tea-colored or dark urine. In the case of statins, certain risk factors have been identified (**Table 11-5**).

Myalgia:
Muscle pain.

Myositis:
Inflammation of the muscle.

Rhabdomyolysis:
A condition resulting from muscle injury that is characterized by muscle breakdown and release of myoglobin into the bloodstream, which can ultimately lead to kidney damage.

Table 11-4 Medications That Can Cause Rhabdomyolysis

Antipsychotics
Antidepressants
Cyclosporine
Sedative hypnotics
Statins
Fibrates
Antihistamines
Illicit drugs (e.g., cocaine)

Data from Huerta-Alardin A, Varon J, Marik P. Bench-to-bedside review: rhabdomyolysis—an overview for clinicians. *Critical Care.* 2005;9:158–169.

Table 11-5 Risk Factors for Statin-Induced Rhabdomyolysis

Patient-Related Factors	Lifestyle-Related Factors
Age (> 80 years old)	Excess alcohol use
CYP 450 isoenzyme polymorphisms	Grapefruit or cranberry juice consumption
Diabetes	Intense exercise
Gender (female)	
Impaired kidney or liver function	
Low body mass index	
Major surgery or trauma	
Untreated hypothyroidism	
Use of CYP 450 substrates or inhibitors	

Data from Sathasivam S, Lecky B. Statin induced myopathy. *BMJ.* 2008;337:a2286.

Cultural Considerations with the Musculoskeletal Exam

A patient's pain experience, perception of pain, and healthcare-seeking practices regarding pain vary based on culture. Healthcare providers are accustomed to asking patients to describe the pain; however, in a culturally diverse society it is important to realize that not all patients will describe pain in the same way. There are a number of descriptive terms that are commonly recognized in the culture of Western medicine to describe various types of pain, such as *sharp*, *dull*, and *stabbing*; in some instances the term used to describe the pain may help the clinician determine the severity or origin of the pain. However, these terms may or may not be used by other cultures, and therefore may not be understood by all patients (Gaston-Johansson, 1990). Conversely, terms used by other cultures to describe pain may not be recognized by the provider (Kaegi, 2004). Use of explanatory models can help the pharmacist better understand how the patient describes the pain, as well as the patient's view and beliefs about pain.

Another consideration is that to express pain or to talk about pain with others is not necessarily an acceptable practice in all cultures (Davidhizar, 2004; Lovering, 2006).

Patients from cultures where it is not customary to discuss pain may choose not to discuss it with a healthcare provider. Depending on the level of trust that the healthcare provider has established with the patient, the patient may share with the provider that he or she is in pain privately. In spite of these differences in regard to discussing pain, it would be appropriate for the healthcare provider to still ask every patient about pain.

In some cultures, the origin of pain may not necessarily coincide with the physiologic origin of pain. For example, the patient may believe that the origin of pain due to an injury or medical condition is due to a violation of a cultural or spiritual belief (Lovering, 2006). In these situations, the patient may not believe that the pain will go away with medical treatment alone. The patient may or may not accept medical treatment for the condition and the pain, but may feel that a visit to a traditional healer or prayer is warranted to truly treat the problem. Some patients may use prayer as a way to cope (Tan, 2005). Asking the patient questions regarding how he or she believes the pain or condition should be treated will provide better insight into how to appropriately treat the patient.

It is also important to note that cultural beliefs regarding pain medication can influence how a patient wishes to manage pain. For example, some cultures may refuse opioid pain medications because of fear of addiction, whereas other cultures may accept opioid pain medications (Lovering, 2006). Prior to making a selection for drug therapy, a discussion with the patient who wishes to use drug therapy should occur. This discussion should include a review of drug therapy classes used to treat the pain and the benefits and risks associated with each class. The patient should then play an integral role in drug therapy selection.

Healthcare providers should also take into consideration their own personal perceptions of pain management and how this can potentially influence how they care for patients' pain (Xue, 2007). If the healthcare provider's views and perceptions of pain differ from those of the patient, this could lead to a breakdown in care. To prevent this, it is important for the healthcare provider to minimize their own personal or cultural judgments regarding the patient's pain experience and how the patient wishes for their pain to be treated.

Example

SZ is a 30-year-old woman recuperating from surgery. She is currently on the general medicine floor at the local hospital. Each shift, the floor nurse comes in to take her vitals and assess her pain score. Each time, SZ reports her pain to be 8 out of 10. Although the physician has included an as-needed order for oxycodone for her pain, SZ continues to refuse to take it, and asks for acetaminophen instead. The nurse is concerned because she knows that acetaminophen will not adequately control her pain. Unsure of what to do, the nurse asks the clinical pharmacist to speak with SZ about her pain management. The pharmacist tells the nurse that SZ refuses to take oxycodone because it is highly addictive, and she would rather suffer than become addicted to a drug and bring shame to her family.

Summary

The pharmacist's assessment of musculoskeletal conditions involves interviewing the patient in addition to performing a limited physical assessment. Because pain can be the presenting symptom for many conditions of both musculoskeletal and nonmusculoskeletal origin, the pharmacist's assessment should include triage to determine if the pain has a nonmusculoskeletal origin, in addition to determining if the musculoskeletal pain is due to a condition or injury that requires medical treatment or if it can be treated using self-care measures. Cultural perceptions and beliefs about pain can influence the patient's healthcare-seeking behavior and treatment methods for pain. As a result, the pharmacist should be sure to take into consideration the patient's beliefs about pain and should include the patient in the decision-making process regarding treatment.

Review Questions

1. A patient approaches you at the pharmacy counter asking for a recommendation to treat her pain associated with a recent injury. She states that 2 days ago while working in the yard she fell off of a ladder and landed on her wrist. She states that the pain is 9 out of 10 on a pain scale. She states that she has been applying ice to the area, but has not had any relief. During your interview with her you begin to wonder if she has broken her wrist, and therefore are wondering if she should be seen by a healthcare provider. What questions would you ask to further determine if she should be seen by her healthcare provider for this injury? What would you look for when inspecting the wrist that would help in making your decision?

2. Explain how the physical exam of a patient with osteoarthritis differs from the physical exam of a patient with rheumatoid arthritis or gouty arthritis.

References

Adis International Limited. Drugs should be considered potential culprits in patients who present with musculoskeletal disorders. *Drugs Ther Perspect.* 2007;23:21–25.

American Academy of Orthopedic Surgeons. Fractures. Available at: http://orthoinfo.aaos .org/topic.cfm?topic=A00139. Accessed August 11, 2013.

American Academy of Orthopedic Surgeons. Sprains and strains: what's the difference? Available at: http://www.orthoinfo.aaos.org/topic.cfm?topic=A00111. Accessed April 28, 2013.

Bannwarth B. Drug-induced musculoskeletal disorders. *Drug Safety.* 2007;30:27–46.

Bannwarth B. Drug-induced rheumatic disorders. *Rev Rhum Engl Ed.* 1996;63:639–647.

Bickley L, Szilagyi P. *Bates' Guide to Physical Examination and History Taking.* 10th ed. Philadelphia, PA: Lippincott Williams & Wilkins; 2009.

Buettner C, Kriegel M, Wells R, Wu J. Statin-induced myopathy and its management. *CML Rheumatol.* 2010;29:105–119.

Callister L. Cultural influences on pain perceptions and behaviors. *Home Health Care Manage Pract.* 2003;15:207–211.

Chumbley E, O'Connor F, Nirschl R. Evaluation of overuse elbow injuries. *Am Fam Physician.* 2000;61:691–700.

Davidhizar R, Giger J. A review of the literature on care of clients in pain who are culturally diverse. *Int Nurs Rev.* 2004;51:47–55.

Davis J, Matteson E. My treatment approach to rheumatoid arthritis. *Mayo Clin Proc.* 2012;87:659–673.

Eggebeen A. Gout: an update. *Am Fam Physician.* 2007;76:801–808, 811–812.

Gaston-Johansson F, Albert M, Fagan E, Zimmerman L. Similarities in pain descriptions of four different ethnic-culture groups. *J Pain Symptom Manage.* 1990;5(2):94–100.

Hawker G, Mian S, Kendzerska T, French M. Measures of adult pain. *Arthritis Care Res.* 2011;63:s240–s252.

Huerta-Alardin A, Varon J, Marik P. Bench-to-bedside review: rhabdomyolysis—an overview for clinicians. *Critical Care.* 2005;9:158–169.

Kaegi L. What color is your pain? Minority Nurse. Available at: http://www.minoritynurse.com/article/what-color-your-pain. Published 2004. Accessed August 22, 2014.

Karnath B, Holden M, Hussain N. Chest pain: differentiating cardiac from noncardiac causes. *Hosp Physician.* 2004;38:24–27.

Lasch K. Culture, pain, and culturally sensitive pain care. *Pain Manag Nurs.* 2000;1:16–22.

Lovering S. Cultural attitudes and beliefs about pain. *J Transcult Nurs.* 2006;17:389–395.

Narayan M. Culture's effects on pain assessment and management. *Am J Nurs.* 2010;110:38–46.

Nayak S, Shiflett S, Eshun S, Levine F. Culture and gender effects in pain beliefs and the prediction of pain tolerance. *Cross-Cult Res.* 2000;34:135–151.

Sathasivam S, Lecky B. Statin induced myopathy. *BMJ.* 2008;337:a2286.

Sinusas K. Osteoarthritis: diagnosis and treatment. *Am Fam Physician.* 2012;85:49–56.

Tan G, Jensen M, Thronby J, Anderson K. Ethnicity, control appraisal, coping, and adjustment to chronic pain among Black and White Americans. *Pain Med.* 2005;6:18–28.

Tomlinson D, Von Baeyer C, Stinson J, Sung L. A systematic review of faces scales for the self-report of pain intensity in children. *Pediatrics.* 2010;126:e1168–e1198.

U.S. Department of Health and Human Services, National Institute of Arthritis and Musculoskeletal and Skin Diseases. What are sprains and strains? Available at: http://www.niams.nih.gov/health_info/sprains_strains/sprains_and_strains_ff.pdf. Accessed April 20, 2013.

Vergne P, Bertin P, Bonnet C, Scotto C, Treves R. Drug-induced rheumatic disorders: Incidence, prevention and management. *Drug Saf.* 2000;23:279–293.

Warren J, Blumbergs P, Thompson P. Rhabdomyolysis: a review. *Muscle Nerve.* 2002; 25:332–347.

Wasserman A. Diagnosis and management of rheumatoid arthritis. *Am Fam Physician.* 2011;84:1245–1252.

Wong-Baker FACES Foundation. Wong-Baker FACES pain rating scale. Available at: http://www.wongbakerfaces.org. Accessed April 27, 2013.

Xue Y, Schulman-Green D, Czaplinski C, Harris D, McCorkle R. Pain attitudes and knowledge among RNs, pharmacists, and physicians on an inpatient oncology service. *Clin J Oncol Nurs.* 2007;11(5):687–695.

Unit IV

The Culturally Competent Care Plan

Putting It All Together

Throughout the course of this text, the reader has learned why a pharmacist should practice culturally competent patient care, how to utilize the patient interview to gather culturally related information that can impact care, and how to conduct patient physical assessments. Unit IV will discuss how each element from the aforementioned chapters can be incorporated into a drug therapy care plan for a patient. Through a series of cases, the reader will be guided through examples on how to develop a culturally competent care plan.

© antishock/Shutterstock, Inc.

Chapter 12

Patient-Centered, Culturally Appropriate Care Models

Carmita A. Coleman, PharmD, MAA
Yolanda M. Hardy, PharmD

LEARNING OBJECTIVE

At the completion of this chapter, the reader should be able to:

1. Integrate findings from cultural explanatory models into the patient care plan.

Introduction

Creating a care plan that is culturally appropriate and takes into consideration the patient's needs, beliefs, and practices regarding management of disease is the goal of providing culturally competent pharmacist patient care. The steps the pharmacist performs in providing patient care can be summarized as follows:

1. Gather information from the patient via patient interview and physical assessment.
2. Identify drug-related problems based on the information gathered.
3. Use this information to formulate a patient care plan.

In order to develop a culturally appropriate care plan, cultural considerations should be integrated into the entire pharmacist care process, starting with the chart review prior to the patient visit and ending with the review of the care plan with the patient.

Integration of Cultural Elements into the Pharmacist Care Process

The patient interview provides a key opportunity to gather information about the patient's condition directly from the patient. Using the core questions, the pharmacist can certainly learn more about the patient's condition; however, the core questions do not allow the clinician to clearly understand the patient's beliefs about the illness or how the patient believes the illness should be treated, if at all. Therefore, an important element in providing

© antishock/Shutterstock, Inc.

culturally appropriate care, and ultimately creating a culturally competent care plan, is to utilize explanatory models to gather more patient-specific information about the illness or condition. The pharmacist can use information obtained from the core questions as well as that obtained as a result of learning about the patient's beliefs to help determine the presence and possibly the cause of drug-related problems.

Performing physical assessment techniques is also a step included in the information-gathering process. Utilization of these techniques will provide the pharmacist with objective information that can further help identify drug-related problems. When performing physical assessment, the pharmacist should be aware of the potential differences in clinical presentation of some conditions in different ethnicities.

Using the gathered information, the pharmacist should then be in a position to identify drug-related problems, as well as the possible reason for the drug-related problems, and develop a culturally competent care plan. When providing culturally competent care, the pharmacist should take into consideration that the cause of the drug-related problem may actually be the result of a patient's belief system. Therefore, the plan should be developed with the patient's input.

Application

The case studies in this section and in the review questions section demonstrate how the aforementioned elements can be incorporated into pharmacist patient care.

Case #1: Kleinman Questions Model

AH is a 45-year-old male who has been admitted to the general medicine floor for hyperglycemia. AH's conversation with the pharmacist follows:

Pharmacist: Hi Mr. H. I am the pharmacist on the floor today. I'd like to ask you a few questions about what brought you here, and then discuss a plan for you and your diabetes. Is that ok?

AH: Sure.

Pharmacist: Thank you. It looks like this is the first time you have been in the hospital for this problem. Can you tell me a little about what symptoms you were having before you came to the hospital?

AH: Well, my usual symptoms. I was feeling really tired, and I kept going to the bathroom to pee. I checked my sugar, and it was 400. I couldn't get it to go down.

Pharmacist: How long has your sugar been this high? When did you notice that you were feeling tired and were going to the bathroom often?

AH: Oh, it started about 3 days ago. That's when I noticed that I was feeling tired and that my sugar was high.

Pharmacist: When your sugar is high like this, and you have these problems, what do you call it?

AH: Oh, I have diabetes. I've had it for a while, but this is just the first time I've been in the hospital for it. I really must have messed up this time.

Pharmacist: What do you mean? What do you think caused this problem?

AH: Well, my diabetes is my punishment from God. I was not a good child, and I think that I'm being punished for that. But it's gotten worse lately.

Pharmacist: Hmmm, what made it worse?

AH: Ever since my wife and I started having problems, my diabetes has been worse. I get so angry with her! That's why I have diabetes, too.

Pharmacist: Why do you think this time you ended up in the hospital? Do you think that this recent episode of your high blood sugars was a punishment?

AH: Yes.

Pharmacist: Why?

AH: I had an argument with my wife. I was so mad. I went to talk to my friends about it, because I knew that it is not good to be angry with your wife. My friends and I went out to eat and I was able to talk about it. We've been going out for the past few nights; you know eating out and drinking a few beers. But being mad is still wrong, so I just have to take my punishment.

Pharmacist: So, tell me, how does this work? You have diabetes because you were bad as a child, and it gets worse when you get angry?

AH: No, well, yes and no. I have diabetes because I was bad. It's my punishment. But it doesn't just flare up when I am angry. I deal with it every day. I have to watch what I eat, because I know that can make my sugars go up, I have to take insulin, and I have to exercise. I have to do those things every day as a constant reminder of how I was as a child.

Pharmacist: Oh, I see. So it sounds like this is something that you will have to deal with for the rest of your life. Is that true?

AH: Maybe. That depends on God. I keep thinking that if I pray and exercise, and eat right, and live a good life, maybe He'll take the diabetes away. But it's hard. Sometimes, my wife just makes me mad, and then I'm angry.

Pharmacist: So, I see that you are on insulin. I'm wondering, what do you think is the best way to treat the diabetes?

AH: I keep thinking that if I pray and exercise, and eat right, and live a good life, maybe He'll take the diabetes away. But it's hard. Sometimes, my wife just makes me mad, and then I'm angry. I still take my medicine, though, but I don't think it really works. I mean, it does something, but I don't think it is what keeps my sugars down. I just think of those insulin shots as just another reminder of my punishment. And if sticking myself is what I have to do to show God I'm sorry, I'll do it. However, I know the shots won't cure me. Only God can do that.

Pharmacist: What other medications are you taking?

AH: I am on insulin, which I take with each meal and at bedtime, baby aspirin, lisinopril, and atorvastatin. I take those every day, too.

Pharmacist: Are you allergic to any medication?

AH: No.

Pharmacist: Has the diabetes caused any problems for you?

AH: I don't think so. I just have to deal with it. Sometimes, if I eat too much for dinner, my wife tells me that my sugars are going to go up, but it doesn't really bother me. I think it may bother her. I think she worries about me and my diabetes.

Pharmacist: What do you fear most about the diabetes and the insulin?

AH: I don't really have a fear about the diabetes or the insulin. My fear is that even though I'm doing everything the best way I know how, that I'm still not going to please God.

Pharmacist: Looking at your blood sugar numbers, the values are pretty high. When the values are this high, increasing the dose of insulin can work to lower the numbers. But tell me, what do you think would make your diabetes better?

AH: Stop arguing with my wife! Ha ha ha! Well, I know that I need to figure out a way to manage my anger. That's what God wants. And I need to keep exercising, praying, and eating right.

Pharmacist: Ok. What are your thoughts about increasing the insulin dose?

AH: Well, I personally wouldn't like it, and like I said, I don't think insulin really does much. I know what I need to do. But I know that having sugars high enough to put me in the hospital is not good, either.

Questions

1. Explain AH's beliefs about why he has diabetes and how it should be managed. How do his beliefs differ from your beliefs? How do they differ from what you learn in pharmacy school about diabetes?

2. Can the pharmacist help AH manage his diabetes? How could his beliefs about diabetes be integrated into your treatment plan for his condition?

Data from Kleinman A. *Patients and Healers in the Context of Culture.* Berkeley: University of California Press; 1980.

The case study shows how the pharmacist can integrate the core questions and the Kleinman questions (1980) into a patient visit. In this example, the pharmacist not only was able to discern pertinent information about what caused the patient's hospital visit, but also was able to learn more about the patient's beliefs on why he has diabetes and what caused this episode of hyperglycemia. Upon reviewing the case, the clinician would conclude that the cause of the patient's hyperglycemia is his period of unhealthy eating and use of alcohol. However, the patient does not directly attribute these behaviors to the cause of his issue. Of note, the patient takes his medication every day as instructed, which would classify him as adherent. However, his motivation for being adherent is related to the fact that he believes that giving himself the injections is something he has to do so show how sorry he is for his past behavior.

The care plan for the management of this patient's hyperglycemic episode should take into consideration both the patient's personal views and the clinician's viewpoints on what is considered standard of care for the management of hyperglycemia; in some instances, this may involve negotiation between the clinician and the patient. An example of a plan for this patient could include the pharmacist working with the patient to ensure that he is eating culturally appropriate foods that will not cause elevations in blood glucose, encouraging prayer, and encouraging exercise. The pharmacist could perhaps refer the patient to someone to further discuss anger management techniques. The pharmacist could also discuss the risks of having elevated blood glucose, and further discuss how insulin can help reduce the blood glucose levels. If the patient's blood glucose has been well controlled in the past, and this elevation is purely based on recent behaviors, perhaps the patient would be amenable to short-term use of a higher dose of insulin. If the patient's blood glucose has been trending upward over a period of time, perhaps further negotiation would be needed to determine if the patient would be willing to increase the insulin dose long term.

As displayed in this case study, neither the core questions nor the explanatory model questions are repeated verbatim from the explanatory models. Patients are very perceptive and can easily determine when the practitioner is using a script to elicit a response. Therefore, practitioners should become comfortable when using a particular model or models, individualizing it to their practice and the situation. Although the questions listed in each model are helpful guides, the pharmacist may need to tailor the questions to help better integrate the questions into the conversation with the patient.

Summary

Culturally appropriate patient care involves not only gathering patient information in a culturally responsive manner, but also developing drug therapy plans that integrate the patient's beliefs and values into disease management. Use of explanatory models that allow the patient to express their thoughts about disease management will assist the pharmacist in making drug therapy decisions that also address the patient's needs and beliefs.

Review Questions

Read the following case study and answer the accompanying questions.

Case #2: BELIEF Model

SJ is a 33-year-old woman who has come to the pharmacy to pick up a new prescription for hypertension. While there, she asks if you could check her blood pressure and recommend a home blood pressure monitoring kit. She states that she was just diagnosed with hypertension. She seems a little anxious about the diagnosis and taking medication for hypertension.

Pharmacist: Hi Ms J. I am the pharmacist. I understand that you would like your blood pressure checked and would like to start checking it at home. I'd like to ask you a few questions about the high blood pressure, and then we can discuss getting a monitor for you.

SJ: Yes, *please.*

Pharmacist: Ok. Well, you were recently told that you have high blood pressure. What do you think caused you to develop high blood pressure?

SJ: Oh, I know why I have it. It's because I am stressed out. I live at home with my mom and my daughter because I lost my job. I've been out of work for 8 months. It's hard to pay my bills, and I feel just horrible that as an adult, I'm relying on my mom to take care of me and my child again. Plus, we don't live in a great neighborhood. I can't take my child out to the park to play because I am afraid something will happen to her. All this has been weighing on my mind. This is why my pressure is up.

Pharmacist: I am certainly sorry to hear about the stressors. You live with your mom. What beliefs do your family members have about high blood pressure? How is your family handling this diagnosis?

SJ: Well, they all have high blood pressure, so the fact that I have it is no big deal to them. Plus, they are all stressed out. It runs in the family. It's like my family can never catch a break. We are always undergoing stressful situations. My mom believes that prayer works, and so every day, she prays and reads the Bible. That keeps her calm and relieves her stress. I think that helps her. I may try it, too.

Pharmacist: Other than prayer, have you considered any other ways to treat the high blood pressure?

SJ: My aunt drinks apple cider vinegar for her blood pressure. I don't think I'm going to do that, because I don't like vinegar.

Pharmacist: Do you have any fears about high blood pressure?

SJ: Sure! My uncle had a stroke after he was diagnosed with high blood pressure. After the stroke, he couldn't work anymore. I don't want that to happen to me. Plus, I don't want my daughter to develop high blood pressure. I'm afraid that if our living situation stays the way it is, she's going to develop it. If I have a stroke, then I may not be able to work at all anymore.

Pharmacist: Ok. I know that you are picking up a medication today for high blood pressure. Do you believe that the medication is the best way to treat the high blood pressure?

SJ: Hmm, not really. The only thing that will fix this is if I get rid of the stress. I don't really trust medications, because they have too many side effects. I'll take it for now, because I know my pressure is high, and maybe it can at least get it down and not worry about it, so then I can focus on finding a job and getting out of my mom's house. Then, when the stress is gone, maybe I won't even need the medicine.

Pharmacist: I can understand that the stress plus this diagnosis can be a lot to deal with. What can I do to help you manage the high blood pressure?

SJ: Well, you've been helpful so far, allowing me to talk to you about this. However, it would really be helpful if you could tell me about some things that I could do to manage this blood pressure without medication. I heard about changing your diet and how that works. If you could tell me about that, I'd

like that. Also, like I said, I don't like taking medicine, so if this medicine is bad for me, or if it causes problems, I need you to tell me.

Questions

1. Explain SJ's beliefs about why she has high blood pressure and how it should be managed. How do her beliefs differ from your beliefs? How do they differ from what you learn in pharmacy school about high blood pressure?

2. Can the pharmacist help SJ manage her high blood pressure? How could her beliefs about high blood pressure be integrated into your treatment plan for her condition?

Data from Dobbie AE, Medrano M, Tysinger J, Olney C. The BELIEF instrument: a preclinical teaching tool to elicit patients' health beliefs. *Fam Med.* 2003;35:316–319.

References

Coronado G, Thompson B, Tejeda S, Godina R. Attitudes and beliefs among Mexican Americans about type 2 diabetes. *J Health Care Poor Underserved.* 2004;15:576–588.

Dobbie AE, Medrano M, Tysinger J, Olney C. The BELIEF instrument: A preclinical teaching tool to elicit patients' health beliefs. *Fam Med.* 2003;35:316–319.

Eisenberg D, Kessler R, Foster C, Norlock F, Calkins D, Delbanco T. Unconventional medicine in the United States—prevalence, costs, and patterns of use. *New Engl J Med.* 1993;328:246–252.

Kleinman A. *Patients and Healers in the Context of Culture.* Berkeley: University of California Press; 1980.

Kleinman AM, Eisenburg L, Good B. Culture, illness, and care: clinical lessons from anthropologic and cross-cultural research. *Ann Internal Med.* 1978;88:251–258.

Kronish I, Leventhal H, Horowitz C. Understanding minority patients' beliefs about hypertension to reduce gaps in communication between patients and clinicians. *J Clin Hypertens.* 2012;14:38–44.

Zaldívar A, Smolowitz J. Perceptions of the importance placed on religion and folk medicine by non-Mexican-American Hispanic adults with diabetes. *Diabetes Educ.* 1994;20:303–306.

Glossary

A

Acanthosis nigricans Brown to black, irregular, velvety hyperpigmentation of the skin often found in folds of the body.

Acculturation To adopt or borrow cultural traits or social patterns from another group.

Acute A condition with sudden onset that may resolve with or without treatment.

Affect Assessed by the mental status examination; how a person expresses a subjectively experienced emotion.

Allergic crease A horizontal line seen across the bridge of the nose that results from repetitively rubbing the tip of the nose in an upward fashion.

Allergic face Facial presentation characterized by facial swelling, darkness around the eyes, and open-mouthed breathing. Patient may also appear fatigued.

Allergic salute The action in which the tip of the nose is rubbed in an upward motion, usually with the palm of the hand.

Allergic shiners Dark circles presenting beneath the eye cavities.

Angina pectoris Discomfort in the chest or adjacent areas due to compromised blood supply to the heart. Also known as angina.

Appearance Assessed by the mental status examination; an individual's dress, grooming, and personal hygiene.

Assimilation The process in which an individual or members of a culture come to resemble those of another culture. Full assimilation occurs when new members of the group are indistinguishable from other members of the group.

Ausculatory gap When assessing blood pressure, the lengthy disappearance of Korotkoff sounds between phase I and phase V.

Auscultation The act of listening to the sounds made by the internal organs with or without a stethoscope, in order to aid in the diagnosis or classification of certain disorders.

B

Behavior Assessed by the mental status examination; particular attention is paid to posture and body movements.

Blood pressure Measure of the force of the blood as it is pushed against the arterial walls.

Bradycardia Resting heart rate less than 60 beats per minute.

Bradypnea Classification that describes a breathing rate considered slower than normal.

C

Chief complaint A major medical or medication-related concern that results in the patient visit. Also considered the purpose of a healthcare visit.

Chronic A condition that presents and lasts for a long period of time. The condition may involve continuous symptoms or may present with intermittent symptoms.

Clinician-centered interview An interview style in which the clinician guides the interview in his or her preferred direction. The clinician's issues of concern may be given priority over the patient's concerns. Patient interaction may be limited.

Cognitive function Assessed by the mental status examination; domains assessed include orientation, attention, memory, learning ability, and problem solving.

Comedones Noninflammatory skin lesion that is the primary sign of acne. It is composed of the dilated hair follicle, skin debris, bacteria, and sebum. May be open or closed. Open comedones are called blackheads; closed comedones are referred to as whiteheads.

Comprehensive interview An interview style with an encompassing focus that typically involves questioning that addresses all areas of a patient's health history.

Contact dermatitis Acute inflammatory condition of the skin caused by an external substance. May be categorized as irritant or allergic. Irritant contact dermatitis is generally caused by exposure to a chemical or irritant that results in skin damage. Allergic contact dermatitis is triggered by an immune response from an allergen.

Cultural competence The ability to provide care that takes into account social, linguistic, and other individual aspects of the patient.

Cultural Formulation Interview (CFI) Instrument introduced in the DSM-5 to account for potential cultural differences in definitions of the mental health problem, perceptions of causes, differences in values regarding coping mechanisms, and help seeking.

Cultural humility An individual's process of self-introspection and reflection in the quest to respect the diverse values, attitudes, beliefs, norms, and traditions of others.

Culturally competent patient care Care that takes into account social, linguistic, and other individual aspects of the patient.

Culturally competent pharmacist patient care The ability to provide appropriate pharmacotherapy treatment that takes into account social, linguistic, and other individual aspects of the patient.

Culture The values, attitudes, beliefs, norms, traditions, language, and so on that are characteristic to a group.

Cyanosis Bluish or grayish coloring seen on the skin near mucous membranes and extremities as a result of poor oxygenation.

D

Diastole Relaxation of the ventricles. During this period, blood is supplied to the heart muscle itself.

Disequilibrium A sensation of feeling off-balance.

Dyspnea Shortness of breath that can indicate breathing difficulties.

E

Eruptions Breaking out of a rash on the skin or a mucous membrane. A drug eruption is an adverse reaction to drug therapy.

Erythema Redness of the skin due to congestion of the superficial capillaries.

Explanatory models A method used when describing a rationale for how or why events happen. Can be utilized during patient interviews to gather an understanding of the patient's beliefs on how or why an illness developed and how and why an illness should be treated.

F

Family history (FH) A listing of medical conditions that members of the patient's family have experienced. Typically includes chronic illnesses that have been experienced by 1st degree relatives or illnesses that cause an increase in hereditary risk of development.

Focused interview An interview style with a limited focus that typically involves questioning limited to the patient's chief complaint, a particular disease state, medication use, or the main reason for the patient visit. Often performed during follow-up appointments.

G

Generalized Describes symptoms that are not limited to one particular area of the body or organ system. Symptoms may affect the entire body.

H

Health disparities Differences in disease incidence and/or prevalence among various cultural groups.

Health equity Attainment of the highest level of health for all people.

Health literacy The ability of an individual to utilize health-related information to make decisions about their own health and health-related issues.

Heart rate Also known as *pulse*. Measure of the number of contractions or beats per minute (bpm).

Heart sounds The sound produced by the heart during the cardiac cycle.

Hemoptysis Expelling blood as a result of coughing.

History of present illness (HPI) A description of the events and symptoms related to the chief complaint.

Hyperpigmentation Unusual darkened area of the skin or nails.

Hypertension A blood pressure equal to or above 140/90 mm Hg.

Hyperventilation Rapid, prolonged, deep breathing that can result from exercise, anxiety, or panic.

I

Inspection Method used in physical assessment that involves looking at a specific body area to assess for abnormalities.

Intermittent claudication A symptom of peripheral artery disease that is characterized by episodes of pain, cramping, and fatigue in one or both legs. It is precipitated by physical exertion and resolves at rest.

Ischemic Heart Disease (IHD) A narrowing of the blood vessels that supply oxygen and blood to the heart.

K

Keloids Elevated, irregular scar of fibrous tissue formed at a site of injury.

Korotkoff sounds Arterial sounds heard when a stethoscope is applied to the brachial artery and pressure is applied from a sphygmomanometer in order to determine the systolic and diastolic blood pressure.

L

Lesions A localized area of damage on an organ or tissue resulting from injury or disease. May be primary or secondary in origin. Primary lesions are caused by a disease process or trauma; secondary lesions occur as a result of primary lesions.

Lightheadedness A sensation of feeling unsteady on one's feet. Sometimes accompanied by the sensation of feeling as if one is about to faint.

Localized Describes symptoms that are limited to one particular area of the body or organ system.

M

Medication history and allergies An account of current and past medication usage. This history should include nonprescription, herbal, and home remedy usage as well as a list of medication-related allergies and the types of reactions caused by the offending agents.

Mental status examination (MSE) Foundational semi-structured interview used to identify patient-specific target symptoms addressed in an individualized treatment plan.

Mood Assessed by the mental status examination; pervasive and sustained emotion.

Moon facies A condition in which the face takes on a full round shape. Can be seen in Cushing's syndrome or as a result of long-term use of high dose corticosteroids.

Murmurs Vibrations resulting from turbulent blood flow within the heart chambers or across the valves.

Myalgia Muscle pain.

Myocardial infarction Occurs when a blood clot has blocked one of the arteries of the heart causing tissue damage.

Myositis Inflammation of the muscle.

P

Palpate To examine by touch or feel.

Past medical history (PMH) A listing of a patient's past and current illnesses, which may also include information regarding onset of illness, year of diagnosis, year of disease resolution, and complications of the disease.

Patient assessment Process used to identify patient problems via evaluation of the patient's subjective reports and objective data.

Patient Health Questionnaire (PHQ) Self-rating scale used by patients as a screening tool for emerging symptoms of depression.

Patient history An account of a patient's entire medical history including, but not limited to, history of medical illness, surgeries, and medication usage.

Patient-centered interview An interview style in which the clinician creates an environment where the patient's concerns are addressed as a high priority. The patient is highly involved and engaged in the interview.

Perceptions Assessed by the mental status examination; characterization of how an individual experiences real external stimuli.

Percussion Method used in physical assessment that involves tapping of a specific body area to assess for abnormalities.

Peripheral neuropathy A condition characterized by nerve damage that presents as sensations of numbness, tingling, and pain in the extremities.

Pharmaceutical care The provision of care that optimizes health outcomes primarily through the use of pharmacotherapeutic agents.

Physical assessment Examination of the body from head to toe using observation, palpation, percussion, and auscultation.

Pitting edema Classification for edema in which an impression is left on the affected area when pressed upon.

Pneumothorax A condition in which air or gas accumulates in the pleural space in the lung cavity.

Presyncope A sensation in which one feels as if he or she will faint.

Primary headache A headache in which the underlying cause is unknown.

Pruritus Itching sensation.

Pseudofolliculitis barbae Razor bumps; persistent irritation caused by shaving.

R

Review of systems (ROS) The portion of the patient history that involves a combination of questioning and physical assessment to assess a patient's health status.

Rhabdomyolysis A condition resulting from muscle injury that is characterized by muscle breakdown and release of myoglobin into the bloodstream, which can ultimately lead to kidney damage.

S

Secondary headache A headache in which the underlying cause is known.

Social history (SH) A description of a patient's nonmedical history. Describes information related to the patient's lifestyle and can include the patient's work history, alcohol and illicit drug use, and dietary patterns.

Speech Assessed by the mental status examination; focus is placed on describing the quantity, rate, and volume of speech as well as the fluency of language and the ability to articulate words.

Sprain An injury resulting from stretching or tearing of ligaments.

Stereotype A broad generalization, positive or negative, that is associated with a specific group of people.

Strain An injury resulting from stretching or tearing of muscle or tendons.

Surgical history A listing of past surgeries. This may also include information regarding the date of the surgery and related surgical complications.

Systole Period of ventricular contraction. The blood is ejected from the heart out into systemic and pulmonic circulation.

T

Tachycardia Heart rate is greater than 100 bpm.

Tachypnea Classification that describes a breathing rate considered faster than normal.

Thought content Assessed by the mental status examination; determination of the presence of unusual thinking or feelings of detachment from reality.

Thought process Assessed by the mental status examination; description of the logical flow, organization, or coherence of ideas and thoughts as expressed by an individual.

Tinea Fungal infection commonly caused by the *Dermatophyte* species.

V

Varicose veins Veins that have become twisted and enlarged, and which may be accompanied by pain.

Vertigo A sensation in which one perceives that his or her surroundings are moving or spinning.

X

Xerosis Abnormal dryness of a body part or tissue, especially of the skin, eye, or mucous membranes.

Index

Note: Page numbers followed by *f* or *t* indicate materials in figures or tables respectively.